TAOIST SECRETS OF
Pregnancy, Birth, *and* Healing Love

"This well-written book by Master Mantak Chia and Marina Dadasheva-Drown includes a fresh perspective and new material dealing with conception, birth, and raising and educating your child. All of these aspects, as well as many exercises, are included here in one book, which includes the authors' wealth of experience and Taoist understanding of how to care for your newborn baby."

WILLIAM U. WEI, COAUTHOR OF *CHI KUNG FOR WOMEN'S HEALTH AND SEXUAL VITALITY*

TAOIST SECRETS OF
Pregnancy, Birth, *and* Healing Love

MANTAK CHIA AND
MARINA DADASHEVA-DROWN

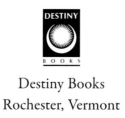

Destiny Books
Rochester, Vermont

One Park Street
Rochester, Vermont 05767
www.DestinyBooks.com

Destiny Books is a division of Inner Traditions International

Copyright © 2022, 2025 by Mantak Chia

Originally published in Thailand in 2022 by Universal Healing Tao Publications under the title *Multi-Orgasmic Birth: Multi-Orgasmic Pregnancy.*

All rights reserved. No part of this book may be reproduced or utilized in any form or by any means, electronic or mechanical, including photocopying, recording, or any information storage and retrieval system, without permission in writing from the publisher. No part of this book may be used or reproduced to train artificial intelligence technologies or systems.

Cataloging-in-Publication Data for this title is available from the Library of Congress

ISBN 979-8-88850-029-3 (print)
ISBN 979-8-88850-030-9 (ebook)

Printed and bound in India by Nutech Print Services

10 9 8 7 6 5 4 3 2 1

Text design and layout by K. Manseau
This book was typeset in Garamond Premier Pro with Present LT Std and Futura Std used as display fonts

To send correspondence to the author of this book, mail a first-class letter to the author c/o Inner Traditions • Bear & Company, One Park Street, Rochester, VT 05767, and we will forward the communication.

Scan the QR code and save 25% at InnerTraditions.com. Browse over 2,000 titles on spirituality, the occult, ancient mysteries, new science, holistic health, and natural medicine.

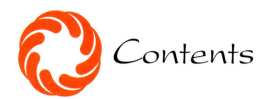
Contents

Acknowledgments	vii
Putting Taoist Secrets of Pregnancy, Birth, and Healing Love into Practice	ix

1	Optimal Vitality and Health	1
2	Knowing Your Own Sexuality	27
3	The Alchemy of Conception	53
4	Pregnancy	85
5	Birth	109
6	Family Care	127
7	The Coming of the Indigo Children	151

Notes	166
Recommended Reading	167
About the Authors	170
The Universal Healing Tao System and Training Center	173
Index	175

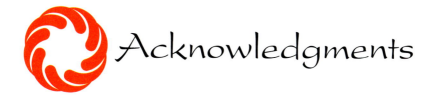

Acknowledgments

This book is dedicated to those who have already given birth and to those who are yet to be participants in this greatest sacrament. The author and coauthor of this book are deeply grateful to those teachers and students who have contributed to this book. We are offering our children and parents the universal energies of love, along with the powerful and pure streams of the Universal Healing Tao and the pure essence of the Tantras.

Special thanks go to the technical creators of this material: The manager of all this work, the one who puts it all together, William Wei, deserves a tip of the hat. Editor and the first reader of individual chapters Colin Campbell Drown deserves credit for his astute contributions. Associates in the complex editorial process are Anastasia Tammen and Anna Novozhilova. Khun Lek leads the great design work of the staff of Tao Garden. Thanks also go to the children of coauthor Marina Dadasheva-Drown: Valentin, Fedor, Igor, Daniel, and Marisha Drown.

And an especially deep bow to all our students and practitioners, for their ideas and creative input concerning human ecology and the importance of conscious conception and freebirth. These ideas and discoveries have been used in this book and are in tune with the latest research by pioneering scientists: geneticist I. Arshavsky, the creator of the doctrine of the biosphere; academician V. Vernadsky; and Chinese scholar and enlightener Lao-tzu. And let us also consider the ideological drivers of India: Mahatma Gandhi, Vivekananda, and the modern humanist, the Fourteenth Dalai Lama.

viii   Acknowledgments

We thank our contemporaries, the people who gave birth and raised beautiful children by practicing the Universal Healing Tao Love. Special gratitude to Dr. Jan Andrew, his wife Fiona, and their beautiful flower of love, daughter Nikita, who have been incredibly open in covering the topic of parenting. As well, big hugs to visionary artists Alex and Alison Grey.

We offer thanks to Igor Charkovsky, who holds an honorary doctorate at the University of California, Berkeley, and is a pioneer of aquatic birth and dynamic developmental training for newborns; as well we thank his associates M. Wagner, D. Pierso, M. Auden, F. Leboye, S. Groff, D. Leonard, L. Ouru, and D. Gamber, who recognize the value of returning to the roots of natural birth. And to Anne Mae Gaskin, Chris Griscom, Sondra Rae, Sheila Kitzinger, Christine Groff, and many other mothers and healers: our deepest gratitude for their sharing their experiences, which have been described in books, articles, and films and are an invaluable contribution toward a new vision for the next generations of humans.

Gratitude goes to our colleagues, for their work on the origins of the physiology and energetics of parenting, and the psychology of pre- and postnatal development of the child: A. Gurevich, Y. Zheleznov, L. Guryanov, L. Kitaeva, and M. Tonenkov, as well as the Brahmin, Anand, Trunov, Kitaev, Sargunu, Kotlar, Lyubimov, Charkovsky, Volodeevich, Drown, Rosenkov, and Ryndich families, who opened the world to the creativity of the emerging generation of Indigo Children.

A huge thank-you to parents who practice the Universal Healing Tao, yoga, internal martial arts, and Tantra, which allow you to responsibly approach the developmental training of your children in a natural way. In particular, thank you for providing us with photos and drawings that depict the practices of the Universal Healing Tao and water birthing methods.

Finally, and not least, and with deepest gratitude, the author and coauthor offer this book about unconditional love to the world.

Putting Taoist Secrets of Pregnancy, Birth, and Healing Love into Practice

The information presented in this book is based on the authors' personal experience and knowledge. The practices described here have been used successfully for thousands of years by Taoists trained through direct personal transmission from teacher to student. Readers should not undertake these practices without receiving personal transmission and training from a certified instructor of the Universal Healing Tao, since certain of these practices, if done improperly, may cause injury or result in health problems. This book is intended as a supplement to individual training by the Universal Healing Tao and as a reference guide for these practices. Anyone who undertakes these practices based on this book alone does so entirely at his or her own risk.

The meditations, practices, and techniques described herein are not intended to be used as an alternative or substitute for professional medical treatment and care. If any readers are suffering from an illness based on physical, mental, or emotional disorders, an appropriate professional health care practitioner or therapist should be consulted. Such problems should be addressed before you start Universal Healing Tao training.

✗ Putting Taoist Secrets into Practice

Neither the Universal Healing Tao nor its staff and instructors are responsible for the consequences of any practice or misuse of the information contained in this book. If the reader undertakes any exercise without strictly following the instructions, notes, and warnings, the responsibility lies solely with the reader.

This book does not attempt to give any medical diagnosis, treatment, prescription, or remedial recommendation in relation to any human disease, ailment, suffering, or physical condition whatsoever.

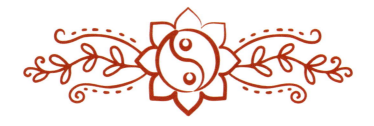

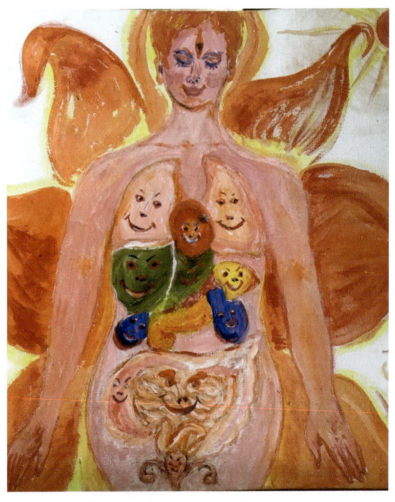

Illustration by Marina Dadasheva-Drown

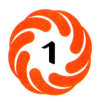

Optimal Vitality and Health

The philosophy enshrined in the Universal Healing Tao system and its practices is designed to work with your body's own self-regulating and healing mechanisms to support your innermost thoughts and feelings. The importance of communicating with your own body allows you to engage creatively with the cosmos. Regular Taoist practice brings harmony in the morning, energy in the afternoon, and tranquility in the evening. The simple truth that a healthy body yields a healthy mind is undeniable. So is the truth that we create good health by building positive emotions in the organs and then spreading these emotions out not only to Earth but to the entire universe! Does this increase our awareness and lead us away from our attachment to the purely material, physical aspect of reality that leads to suffering? Of course it does! And for those couples who want to bring new life into the world, Taoist practice increases their self-confidence and extends their ability to instill Healing Love, the very essence of the Tao, in the next generation, thereby creating the basis for harmonious family relationships and ultimately a harmonious world.

The Tao teaches us how to preserve our energy, how to transform it, and how to keep it in our bodies by directing our sexual energy upward, toward our higher, spiritual chakras. If you don't know how

2 Optimal Vitality and Health

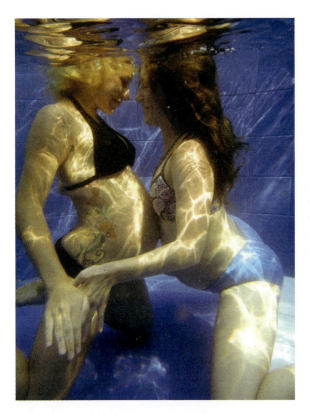

Fig. 1.1. Taoist practice increases self-confidence and extends the ability to instill Healing Love in the next generation.

to do this, your vital life-force energy basically ends up going to waste. Take monks and nuns who turn away from the world, saying, "I am holy, I am not of this world." A monk closes his eyes and sees no evil, covers his ears and hears no evil, and places his hands over his mouth and speaks no evil. And he also covers his sex organs so they will do no evil. People who choose a monastic life ultimately say no to sex. The rest of us have no idea what life without sex is like for them. Maybe they take this sexual energy and move it upward in their bodies. Or maybe we should think of them as supermen and superwomen for their superpower of not having or wanting sex? Maybe, unlike the rest of us, monks do not produce any sperm, and nuns cease to menstruate. Of course this cannot possibly be the case—monks still produce sperm, and nuns still have their eggs and continue to menstruate. They cannot deny the sexual part of their being or wish it away. Which is precisely the reason why we sometimes hear about monks who secretly have sex.

We've all heard about priests in the West who not only have sex but, as we now know, do so with children, because the sexual part of their nature cannot be stilled. Understanding the sexual nature of our being is thus the key to our transformation.

The transformation we're talking about is nothing less than a change and a renewal of our DNA. This requires sex, orgasm, love, and compassion, as well as synchronizing with the very heartbeat of Mother Earth. The first love vibration we get is from the cells of our father and our mother, who, when aroused, made love and had an orgasm because of their love and compassion. Sex organs to sex organs. They loved each other and wanted to create more love. The man's best energy is directed toward his sperm, and the woman's best energy is directed toward her eggs. This energy, the energy of love, multiplies and radiates. We can literally see this when we look at a sex cell: it can multiply over and over, up to fifty trillion times. This is some incredible power!

Science says the human body completely changes its cells every seven years, but the process of duplicating the information for future cells happens continually. This explains how such feelings as anger and hatred can end up lasting for many, many years. The only thing that can wipe these feelings away is arousal, orgasm, love, and compassion. And this is exactly what happens when a woman and a man make love, and the man passes his primal energy to his sperm, and the woman passes her original force to her egg. Tremendous power and energy occurs as a result of the sperm's primal force and the egg's original force meeting.

This original, primal force is what draws energy in from the universe, and it is deposited in the very first cell we manifest. It is only later that the soul is drawn into the newly created body, followed by the spirit (sometimes called the subconscious). When all these powerful forces come together, they produce a sound, a vibration. This is the truest sound of life: the beginning of the human pulse. Mere weeks within conception there is already a heartbeat. We take our first breath the moment we emerge from the womb. The beating of the heart that gives us our pulse is forever out of our conscious control, the same way that breathing is unconscious and part of the true sounds of life.

4 Optimal Vitality and Health

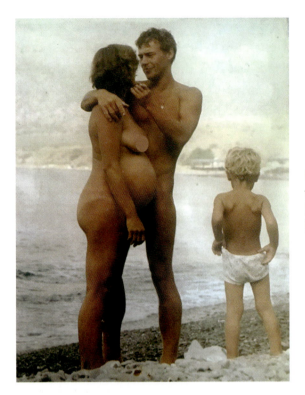

Fig. 1.2. The first love vibration we get is from the cells of our father and our mother.

Our brain never stops controlling our breathing, not even when we are asleep, floating between our conscious and our subconscious mind. It is well-known that our subconscious can help us achieve our goals. It usually goes like this: you set a goal, you pray for it, you believe in it. Through the process of setting the goal and praying for its realization, you're directing your energy from your conscious mind to your subconscious mind. But to actually realize your goal, you need that primal force, and you need a lot of it; if there isn't enough, you simply cannot achieve what you've set out to achieve. Those of us who don't have enough of that primal force barely have enough energy to sleep, or else they pass on because their subconscious simply does not have the energy to continue.

This primal force, known as *chi* or *prana*, controls the nervous system and all the bodily functions. The mind must get to work to generate enough energy so that this primal force can pass from the conscious to the subconscious. Our heartbeat, breath, digestion, absorption, and elimination—indeed, all the physical functions of the body—require direction from the subconscious. One quarter of all our original life force that we receive at birth goes to our kidneys and is stored there for any possible emergencies. For those who do not have a lot of energy to begin with, there will be very little reserves, if any at all, for emergencies. Adrenaline will kick in and the fight-or-flight mode will activate, allowing you to run very fast away from danger and toward safety, toward life. But this will not ensure your survival without wisdom and intelligence playing their part.

When there is no more energy left in the kidneys, it means the end. In this moment of truth, the soul and spirit will depart because there will not be enough energy to do what's needed to support the physical body. When fighting for their lives, our ancient ancestors would retreat into caves to survive, and the fight-or-flight chemical adrenaline served them well. Eventually, however, humans turned to studying the functions of the body, which in turn prompted the rise of Chinese medicine, acupuncture, and other healing modalities. At that time there was no thought of the afterlife, of heaven and its rewards and hell with its punishments. These ancient Taoists instead looked at the relationship between humans and nature and looked at the universe as a whole. They eventually went on to study human consciousness and the subconscious, the spirit and the soul, which they believed a person could learn to master. They discovered and taught practices that helped us improve our physical and spiritual health, without imposing fear and the concept of hell and punishment, concepts that go back many generations and have been imposed on many of us since early childhood.

Sexual energy is the strongest power we humans possess, and like any powerful tool out there, it can help us or cause us problems. Fire, when handled with care, helps us cook our food and warm our home. But if mistreated, it can easily burn our house down and even burn whole cities to the ground.

The Tao is concerned with sexual and eliminative organs and their connection to the emotions. There's also a connection between these and all the other organs, which fall into the following categories:

Yin: Heart, lungs, spleen, pancreas, liver, and kidneys
Yang: Small intestine, Triple Warmer, large intestine, gallbladder, and urinary bladder

Each of our organs contains energy, which gets depleted when we experience strong negative emotions. Hatred and impatience drain the heart. Worry and anxiety drain the spleen and the pancreas. Sadness and grief drain the energy of the lungs. Fear, phobias, and trauma drain the kidneys. Anger and jealousy drain the liver. All of these energies drained from our organs end up escaping through the anus, and in women this can also happen through the cervix. This is why the Tao is concerned with having control over our sexual desire and

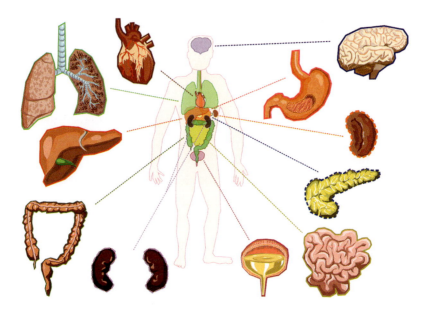

Fig. 1.3. The organs of the human body. The lungs supply oxygen and remove CO_2; the heart pumps blood to bring oxygen and nutrients to the entire body and to remove CO_2 and toxic waste; the liver and kidneys detox blood; the nervous and endocrine systems regulate the metabolism; the immune system protects us against viruses, bacteria, and foreign matter; and the musculoskeletal system supports the body's structure and the placement of the organs.

especially our emotions, so that this draining of vital energy from the organs can be prevented. If you do not take care of your organs, they cannot take care of you. And a problem with just one organ can breed issues in others.

So study human anatomy! The key to cultivating health in your organs is knowing what they look like and where they're located. The Tao asks, Is it your entire sacred human body that you want to enhance, or merely the superficial aspects of your body so that you'll look good in yoga pants? You must get to know the organs and hold their images in your mind. Enlightenment is right here, located in the powerful sex organs! Look at them and smile at them.

REJUVENATING EXERCISES FOR MEN AND WOMEN

The Tao says that if you continue to lose energy through your sex organs and through your anus, you will soon be depleted of the vital life force.

For women, the primal energy drains out through the cervix and vagina. Look at your vagina, cervix, and anus. Smile at your ovaries and your uterus. Lightly contract your anus and vagina and close the mouth of your cervix. Visualize it lightly closing. For men, it's the opening of the penis and the anus that need to be closed. The prostate is another organ that must be given attention, as it can cause a lot of problems as a man ages. The prostate is just below the bladder. Look at the penis, the prostate, and the anus. Lightly close the opening of the penis and contract your anus. Touch your pubic bone just below the prostate. Your prostate has three holes in it, and they must be closed lightly as well. When you do this, the Three Yin Channels are closed. Pull the drained energy back into the organs. Press the tongue up to the roof of your mouth to complete the circuit. See the violet light of the universe, the light of wisdom. Let feelings of love, joy, and happiness come over you. Once you learn how to do this, you will have a lot more energy.

Einstein's theory of special relativity is understood by Taoists as follows:

$$E = mc^2$$

where

$$E = chi$$

$$m = mass$$

c^2 = speed of light squared (in the human body, this is the creative element of fire)

This is the formula for transforming mass into energy, and this is something we can do in our own bodies. Of the five elements—earth, air, fire, water, and metal—it is the element of fire that is employed in the ultimate creative act of human sexuality. It is also what we are activating when we do the Abdominal Breathing exercise, described below.

Abdominal Breathing

Abdominal Breathing is the basic breathing technique used in many of the exercises of the Universal Healing Tao. It draws chi into the navel center, or lower tan tien, which is considered our main energy storage center, or biobattery. This is the location of the enteric nervous system, which is part of the autonomic nervous system that is sometimes called the "second brain." This center plays an essential role in regulating the body's functions. It's a rich source of neurochemicals that affect mood and well-being.

There are two aspects to this exercise: simple abdominal breathing, and reverse abdominal breathing.

1. Stand with your feet shoulder-width apart, toes pointed straight forward. Keep your shoulders relaxed, spine straight, chest slightly sunk, knees slightly bent, and tailbone slightly tucked (imagine that you started sitting on a chair and then changed your mind).

Optimal Vitality and Health 9

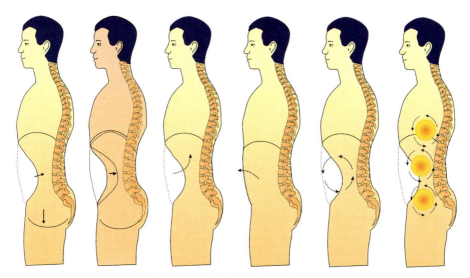

Fig. 1.4. Abdominal Breathing.
Suction in the abdomen draws chi into this area.

2. Take a deep breath, and as you let it out, relax. Repeat a few times. Now bring your attention to your abdominal area. Smile into your body.
3. Focus on your navel and imagine there is a balloon right behind it. As you inhale, expand this balloon with a longer breath so that your abdomen expands.
4. As you exhale, shrink this balloon so that your navel is pulled inward toward the spine. The exhalation should be shorter than the inhalation.
5. Repeat the whole sequence of Abdominal Breathing either 9, 18, 27, or 36 times, then rest. Once you are comfortable with this basic form of abdominal breathing, proceed to the next step.
6. Now you will do reverse abdominal breathing. This means that you will pull your navel toward your spine on the inhalation and relax your abdomen on the exhalation.
7. Repeat 9 times. Pay attention to how you feel. When this way of breathing becomes comfortable, you can do 18, 27, or 36 repetitions.
8. Now go back to normal abdominal breathing again. Inhale and expand your abdomen, then exhale all the air out, pulling your

navel toward your spine as you exhale. Imagine that your navel is touching your spine. In this position, on the end of the exhale, you will hold your breath for a few seconds while visualizing the suction in your abdomen pulling chi in. Then, inhale and relax your abdomen. Repeat 9, 18, 27, or 36 times.
9. Finish the practice by smiling and taking a few deep, relaxing breaths. With practice you will develop a state of wonderful lightness and ease of breathing with your entire body.

For Men

Sending Fire to the Genitals

For men, the primary focus of energy is the testicles. What we want to do is move fire down to the testicles, and this fire will in turn transform the energy there to reinvigorate the testicles.

The palm of a human hand is special; it can gather and channel a lot of energy, and you can activate this energy by rubbing both of your hands together. Do this before beginning this practice.

1. Massage and squeeze the testicles; there may be some painful sensation.
2. Place one hand over your testicles and another one on your kidneys. Kidneys are directly affected by ejaculation; an excess amount of it will be harmful to your kidneys.
3. Your hands hold the chi energy, so this exercise will help the testicles to send the energy up to the kidneys.

For Women

Warming the Breasts

Nature has endowed a woman's body with the ability to conceive and give birth; once a month it prepares for the fertilization of an egg, whether the woman wants a child or not. The breasts become energized to produce milk. As a result, the uterus receives the best high-quality energy for a good conception. If conception does not happen, the body ends up cleaning out the uterus and all that energy gets wasted—unless, of course, a woman knows how to prevent this loss of valuable chi by engaging Taoist practices such as this one. We lose so much energy without even knowing it, simply by doing nothing with it. This wasted energy causes a problem for the breasts, since all that preparation for milk production ends up being cut short.

This breast massage creates fire. You should feel your breasts warming up, like the sun shining on the water, creating steam. Before beginning this practice, activate this energy by rubbing both of your hands together to stimulate chi.

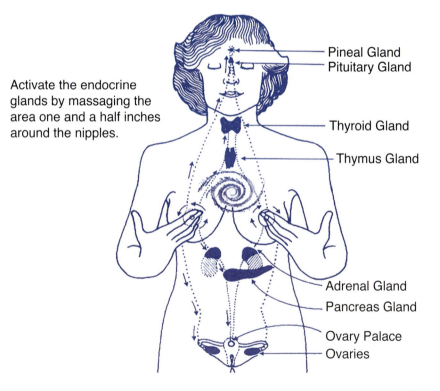

Fig. 1.5. Breast massage can invigorate and firm the breasts and replenish the skin of the chest, neck, and shoulders.

1. Move your breath to your ovaries and uterus.
2. Hold your palms under your breasts and gently circle inward. Use massage oil if you like and make 9 inward circles. Then reverse direction and make 9 outward circles.
3. Massage your nipples, which activates contractions in the uterus. Then massage down with tiny circular movements along the line that connects your nipples to your public bone.
4. Make sure that your liver and spleen are enriched with blood, as they both are affected by menstrual bleeding. To do this, hold one of your breasts and place the other hand over your spleen; same with your liver. Then place both hands over your liver and your spleen; this allows the energy of the breasts to revitalize the liver and the spleen. While performing this massage, imagine the sun shining on water. Feel the energy moving through your sacrum and upward, to revitalize your brain, or upper tan tien. You can also direct this energy to any other organ that needs healing.
5. Finish by holding your breasts and gently shaking them. Remember to smile inwardly throughout this exercise.

Testicle Breathing and Ovarian Breathing

Taoist practices such as those described here are all based on the principle that there is a connection between the conscious mind and the subconscious. These are powerful practices that transform the leakage of chi that inevitably happens in men through ejaculation and in women through menstruation. In addition to the aforementioned practices, very good results can also be achieved with the techniques of Testicle Breathing for men and Ovarian Breathing for women.

1. Standing upright, begin with the Abdominal Breathing exercise, described earlier in this chapter.
2. Once you're comfortable with this form of breathing, contract your pelvic floor muscle. At this point, women should feel their ovaries and uterus lifting up; men will feel the same upward lift in their testicles.

3. While continuing abdominal breathing, repeat this pelvic contraction 9 times. Pay attention to how you feel. Once this way of breathing becomes comfortable, you can do 18, 27, or 36 rounds.
4. As you practice, you'll begin to notice a sensation in your brain, the upper tan tien. At that point pull your perineum up. Men should also focus on their prostate gland and feel it lifting. As you pull your pelvic floor muscles up, you will start to feel your chi moving.

Activating the Three Fires

In addition to their physiological roles, the organs have energetic roles. These are known as the three fires, or tan tien. These are the major energy centers for storing chi.

The upper tan tien, or brain, cannot store too much energy because it can easily overheat. Modern life causes people to focus outwardly and consume too much negative information, which generates a lot of heat in

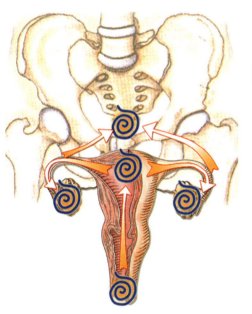

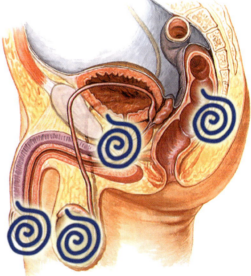

Fig. 1.6. Ovarian Breathing moves chi throughout the female reproductive organs.

Fig. 1.7. Testicle Breathing moves chi throughout the male reproductive organs.

the brain, creating conditions for mental imbalance. However, this center can also be used to connect to the vast energy available in the universe.

The middle tan tien, or heart, also cannot store too much energy because it too easily overheats. It is better used to multiply one's emotional energy and radiate it out to connect to other people. Taoists maintain that the heart is connected to the unconditional love available throughout the universe.

It is the lower tan tien, or the abdominal center, that serves as the body's main biobattery; it stores large amounts of energy to supply the body's needs.

When negative energy gets stuck in any (or all) of these three centers, it causes any number of physical and emotional problems, meaning the brain, heart, and gut are disconnected and have forgotten how to work together. Taoist practice teaches us that it is very important to bring excess heat down from the brain and the heart to the main biobattery, the lower tan tien. This means we must have a clear understanding of the location of the three major fires and know how to bring the excess heat down.

1. The upper tan tien is located in the center of the brain. Touch your third eye, the point between your eyebrows, and project chi all the way to the back of your skull. Touch the tops of your ears and project chi through the imaginary line connecting your ears. Then draw an imaginary line from the crown to the perineum.

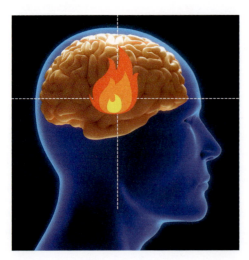

Fig. 1.8. The upper tan tien (brain) fire

Optimal Vitality and Health 15

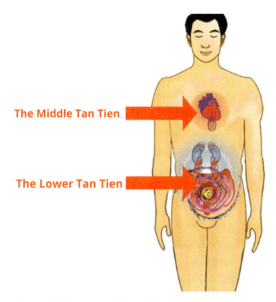

Fig. 1.9. The middle tan tien (heart) fire and lower tan tien (abdominal) fire

2. Breathe and smile into the upper fire.
3. The middle tan tien, or heart fire, can be located by drawing a line from a point located one inch above the tip of the sternum on the midline, to the middle section of the vertebral column, between the lumbar and the cervical vertebra, and then finding its intersection with the line that goes from the crown to the perineum.
4. Breathe and smile into the middle fire.
5. The lower tan tien, or navel center, can be located by drawing an imaginary line from the navel to the Door of Life, which is the point on the spine opposite the navel. This fire is located below the intersection, in a triangular space between the navel or Door of Life (which is also the kidney center) and the sexual center.
6. Breathe and smile into the lower fire.

Your sacrum and pubic bone work together to move chi through your body. This is the core practice. If you do not exercise this area enough and you eat a lot or incorrectly, there is a very high risk of problems with digestion. To achieve good results, these practices must be put to use—in other words, this is a training, and training requires self-discipline. You must actually do these practices!

The Million Dollar Point for Men

In men, the space between the anus and the entire structure of the male sexual organs is a powerful acupressure point. This point is considered so important that it has been called the "Million Dollar point." Massaging this point helps activate male sexual energy flow and removes blockages.*

1. To locate this spot on your body, first find your anus. Just in front of it you will find a dip between two bones; press there with your middle finger.
2. Continue this practice every day until this point opens, which will feel like the point is softening to your touch. Ensuring that this point is open is crucial for Taoist energy work, as this is the root of the core channel in men.
3. After regularly practicing this technique, the moment you notice energy moving up in your body, turn your gaze inward and upward and you will see in your mind's eye a little green light. This is your signal.
4. Roll your eyes up and back inside your head. Pull your breath up as you inhale and contract. Exhale.
5. Repeat this breathing process 9 times. Feel a line running up from your perineum into your skull. This energy goes up and then to all the organs of the body. Whenever you feel aroused, you need to pull this arousal energy up to your upper tan tien, or brain, or to one of your organs.
6. Move the chi from your coccyx to your brain, from the bottom to the top. Then rest.
7. Shake your body out a little and relax.

---

*Master Chia was the first to write about this point in his book *Taoist Secrets of Love: Cultivating Male Sexual Energy* (Aurora Press, 2016).

Learn these "routes," as they are so important: from the earth to the perineum, from the anus and organs up to the brain.

SMILING JADE EGG FOR WOMEN

Let's now consider the Smiling Jade Egg exercise as a training for women that increases sexual energy, enhances partner sex, and is also a great preparation for motherhood. Taoist teachers do not suggest starting this training, which is of a more intimate nature, without the guidance of a Universal Healing Tao instructor. This meditative genital exercise for women has no contraindications if the woman is comfortable with her sexuality and her body. If in doubt, it is best to consult a specialist about the health of the flora and any possible infections in the birth canal.

The most beautiful material for meditative erotic creativity is jade, a stone connected to the elements of water and earth whose energies

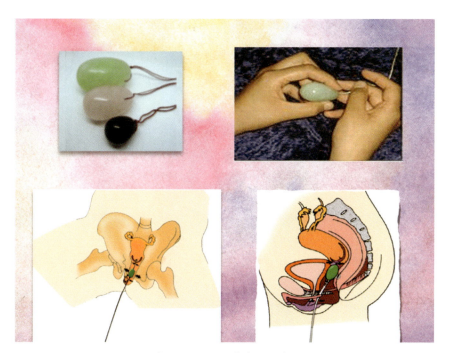

Fig. 1.10. Moving the egg up and down, the Yoni Egg practice

18 Optimal Vitality and Health

promote peace, fertility, healing, beauty, and protection. Jade comes in different colors; the color should be chosen to match the taste and mood of the woman. This practice moves energy in the sacred space of the vagina and has many benefits, among them:

- Better circulation and flow through mindfulness, helping to release toxins and any negative energy
- Energy clearing through the nature of the stone, jade, which absorbs negative energy
- Hydration of connective tissues through squeezing and releasing
- Helps the brain stay vibrant due to the action of moving energy up the spine

There are special jade eggs for this purpose that have holes at the thinner end, where you can lace a string. The size and shape of the egg you choose should correspond to the shape of your vagina, which is approximately the size of your mouth cavity, as the egg should be able to be very conveniently placed in your mouth, posing no inter-ference with the gums and teeth when closing your lips. All women need to love their bodies and know the features of their "secret cave," the yoni—the depth, elasticity, and strength of its ring of muscles. It is equally important to measure with your thumb the length of the perineum, the "island" between the anus and the outer vagina. Using your finger, you can also determine the elasticity of your "secret gate," the outer ring muscle, by placing it a centimeter in, pressing down toward the anus and pulling back. This exercise is helpful for a woman in preparation for pregnancy and childbirth. In vaginal massage (as well as in the ritual study of the male prostate), it is important to moisten your finger with saliva or lubricate it with pure coconut or castor oil.

After determining the size and shape of your vagina, set the place and time for daily or periodic sessions with your jade egg. Respect the intimate nature of this exercise and cultivate a positive attitude. The best time is in the morning, and as to place, choose one that is

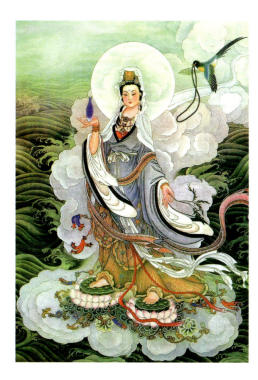

Fig. 1.11. Kuan Yin is the female bodhisattva of compassion.

associated with a spiritual presence to help create the mood. Statues of goddesses or other divine female figures adorned with a string of your beads or pearls or crystals are appropriate, as their presence purifies the mind and inspires thoughts of love and eroticism. In Chinese culture there's a lot of respect for Kuan Yin, one of the highest female manifestations of the Buddha. The Egyptian goddess Sekhmet, sometimes shown breast-feeding her infant son, is another possibility, as are the Hindu goddesses Lakshmi, Parvati, and Radha. Many women gravitate to Ganesha, the herald of love, forgiveness, eroticism, and fertility. The image chosen should relate to a woman's sense of eroticism.

Yoni Egg Practice

1. Before using your egg, wash it thoroughly with soap and hot, clean water or your own warm urine. Be sure to wash the egg after using it as well, and store it in a clean, dry place, and consider placing it in the sunlight or moonlight to charge its energy.

2. If your stone comes with a string, replace it with dental floss, which you will discard after each use. The string should be the length of your arm from your fingertips to your elbow. Fold the floss in half and thread the folded end through the hole in the egg. You should have a loop on one end and two loose ends on the other end. Thread the loose ends through the loop and let it tighten, so the egg is secure. Set it aside.

3. Begin by meditating in a comfortable lotus or diamond position, heels under the buttocks. The palms of your hands are open and ready to be filled with cosmic or solar/lunar energies.

4. Imagine yourself as a goddess and caress your breasts, arousing your nipples and your consciousness. To be effective, a meditation requires that you form a clear intention and remain immersed in the meditation. When we know exactly why we engage in this or that practice, life processes in the brain are stimulated thanks to the hippocampus, which contributes to the concentration in the execution of the intention.

5. As you meditate, place your hands on your heart and smile through your third eye to your thymus, located between the upper part of your breasts. Feel your heart opening like a loving lotus, then send this smile to your uterus, warming it with a stream of sunlight. The feeling of loving attention will penetrate the cells of your body and your consciousness. The palms of your hands slide over to your nipples to warm them. Rotate your index fingers around them, extending the range of motion, revealing two fragrant flowers; gently press on these swollen pistils and direct your sensuality to your ovaries, visualizing the Milky Way, arousing the ovaries.

6. Return to your breasts and gently massage them. Then descend to the liver and spleen, and place your hands over those organs, sending light and color to them—a sparkling, pastel green and golden yellow light. Imagine flowers blooming in these shades at the level of these organs. Mentally connect them with your cervix and ovaries, filling them as well with the energy of these colors.

7. Shake off any excess heat from your palms or rub them together to activate chi and warm them up even more.

Optimal Vitality and Health **21**

8. Lower your third eye and visualize your blue, luminous kidneys as the buds of magnificent water lotuses opening as you continue the circular massage of your breasts, their energy connecting with the ovaries and the clitoris. Then place your palms over the area of your ovaries (your thumbs are touching on the navel, and where the pinkies meet are the ovaries).

9. Softly contract your perineum, release the energy there, and pull it up into your internal sex organs. Pink and white lotuses in the ovaries stimulate kundalini energy. One hand rises to the heart, the other covers the pubis and the labia, connecting spiritual and physical arousals.

10. At this point, insert the jade egg into your yoni, wide end of the egg first. It is good to use mantras or chant while you do so. If you're just starting to learn this sacrament, then do this while lying on your back, with bent knees and feet resting comfortably near your buttocks. This is the best position for relaxing the pelvic muscles and inserting the egg through your sacred gate into your vagina.

11. Flex your yoni muscles. The main point is to feel the egg, to which you've previously attached the length of floss (outlined in step number 2 above). The muscles are trained by squeezing the larger end of the egg at the uppermost part of your vagina while your fingers are pulling at the thread as if trying to pull the egg out, creating a counterforce. This exercise can be varied by using different breathing techniques; for example, holding your breath at the point of tightening of the muscles and then inhaling at their relaxation.

12. At the end of the session with the egg it is important that you shoot it out of your vagina using your muscles—do not pull it out by the string!

13. Don't forget to smile inwardly throughout this entire practice.

In preparation for conception we do not advise engaging in bodybuilding or strenuous workouts. The idea of training in the Taoist sense is to give the muscles elasticity and firmness. Playing the muscles like a musical instrument, we excite the libido, keep the sperm in the cervix and in the

22 Optimal Vitality and Health

uterus, where it is washed by the woman's ejaculative fluids of amrita and pushes the sperm up into the fallopian tubes, where an egg will merge with a successful sperm. It is necessary to know that the readiness for ovulation is created by the vibration of many eggs, which create the possibility for a single egg saturated with hormones to be implanted in the uterus after conception. The epithelium, the protective layer of cells that line hollow organs and glands, is the "soil of the uterus," a fertile, vitamin-saturated soil that regenerates from one menstrual cycle to another. Every month, all our organs and the body as a whole send enormous energy potentials to our reproductive organs for future fertilization. This creates colostrum in the breasts and enough epithelium in the uterus. Every month a woman loses one or more deenergized eggs, along with menstrual blood and unused colostrum. Every woman should do her best to minimize blood loss, focusing on her emotional comfort, returning energy to the organs, and absorbing any unused colostrum.

Breast massage relieves tension, and the transformation of menstrual blood into vitality nourishes the organs and creates the impulse for new, healthy ovulation. The Microcosmic Orbit, described in chapter 2, along with the energy pulsations of the sexual muscles, raises chi up the spine and brings it down the front canal to the Hui Yin region, located at the very root of the torso, at the center of the pelvic floor, a half-inch in front of the anus. There it holds the information in the storage unit, the bladder, where it crystallizes and fills the memory code with a desire for conscious conception, or conversely, for transformation into the life force to prevent unwanted fertilization. Thought, intention, and energy flow create the possibility for conception or its prevention. It is very important as well that those who are striving to have children think about what needs to be changed for the better in themselves so that this "something," improved and more honest, will help to improve life for many generations on Earth.

ATTENDING TO YOUR BONES

Finally, we strongly advise women as well as men to tap bamboo hitters along the channels of their bodies. If bamboo sticks aren't readily available, tapping can be performed with the palms of the hands or loose fists. The Taoist practice of Nei Kung* rejuvenates bone marrow and stimulates vital processes in your body and removes toxins. All Taoist practices are based on the bone system. The palace of bone marrow is situated in our hip bones, connected with the ligament psoas muscles. Since a woman bears a child in her belly, it is very important to use the soft tapping between these bones, which support the baby's "house." All the bones of the body are tapped—arms, shoulders, and cervical, cranial, and facial (light, fast tapping) bones.

On the sternum and ribs we affect the vibrations of the fasciae in the nearby organs. Moving down to the pelvic area, do not forget the pubic bone, coccyx, and the entire sacral area. Since our basic energy is sexual, in many Taoist healing practices the handle of a bamboo hitter is used to gently tap at the crotch area from the anus to the pubis. Men use their other hand to grab and lift the external genitals. Women get a particularly pleasant and exciting sensation that can rise up like a raging torrent. These practices are very helpful in preparation for pregnancy. They should be continued even in pregnancy from the fourth to the fifth month when the sexual life is possibly not very active, and the hip part of the woman's body needs good blood flow and lymph circulation. Before and after tapping it is good to rub the area between the legs until it's warmed up; this contributes to the elasticity of the ligaments. All these practices help a woman bear the child joyfully and minimize pain in childbirth, and some women might even give birth in the sensation of a powerful orgasm.

 ## Tapping for Bone Health

Taoists believe that enhancing bone health is necessary to keep the body aligned and supported, as well as to activate chi throughout the body.

---

*See Master Chia's book *Bone Marrow Nei Kung: Taoist Techniques for Rejuvenating the Blood and Bone* (Destiny Books, 2006).

24   Optimal Vitality and Health

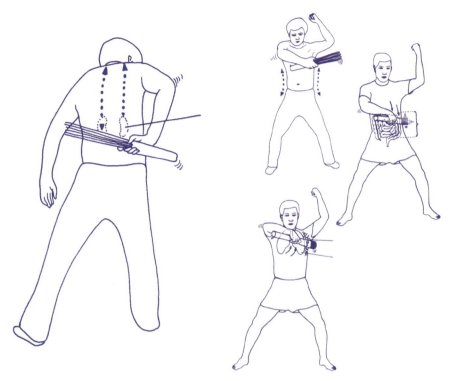

Fig. 1.12. Tapping with a bamboo hitter on all the points on the arms, torso, and legs

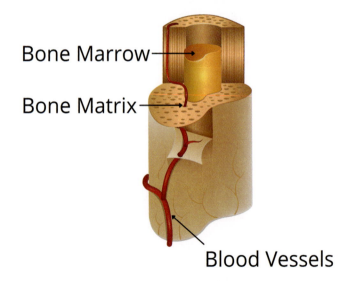

Fig. 1.13. Inner structure of a bone

1. Begin by standing correctly: feet shoulder-width apart, toes pointed straight forward. Keep your shoulders relaxed, spine straight, chest slightly sunk, knees slightly bent, and tailbone slightly tucked (imagine that you started sitting down on a chair and then changed your mind).
2. Take a deep breath and as you let it out, relax. Send a smile and a ray of healing sunshine to any areas that hurt, and the pain will dissipate. Starting at the feet, travel up the body through its bone structure, moving and sending your smile and sunshine energy everywhere.
3. Focus on your joints and shake them vigorously for 1 to 2 minutes, from head to toes, while remaining pleasantly relaxed.
4. Stop and stand still, noticing the movement of chi in your body.
5. Warm the palms of your hands by rubbing them together and massage and tap the bones. Direct energy to any spot that needs healing.

There is always a danger that sexual arousal will lead to temptations. Advertising knows all about the strength of sexual arousal—advertisers constantly project sexual images to attract our attention, and boom! Our wallets and purses open. They have us under a spell to make us buy whatever they are selling. We are captured by our senses—my eyes desire, my nose desires, my ears desire, my mouth desires. You cannot control these desires unless you learn how to transform your sexual energy. So do these basic practices! As you gain experience with them, you will find yourself controlling your anus and your vagina or penis. Once you have learned how to prevent energy leakages in these important points, you will start gaining control of your sexual desires and sexual temptations to create balance and optimal vitality.

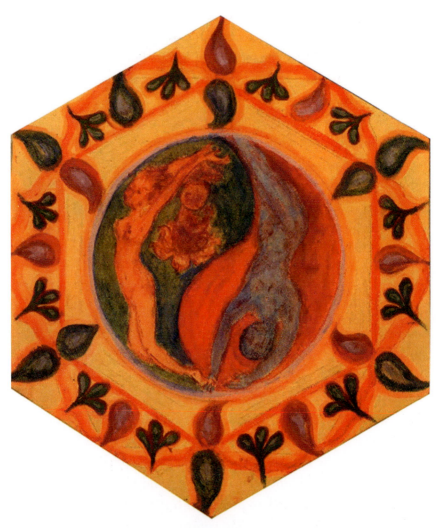

Illustration by Marina Dadasheva-Drown

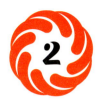

Knowing Your Own Sexuality

Did the universe intend for us to be conceived, nurtured, and born in love, vibrating with the most precious and beautiful abilities of our souls and bodies? Many ancient cultures believed this to be so, as stated in the Vedas, the Celtic runes, and the entire Taoist culture of Healing Love, which is based on a human being's basic energies and their natural transformative capabilities. We also find the same ideas in various branches of Tantra. In the very conception and birth of a person, gradual sexual development is taking place, and it is only enriched by love.

Balance is what preserves life on Earth. Nature and the Divine have provided all that is necessary to help us find and keep that balance. All conflicts arise from failure to expand our consciousness, as consciousness leads to knowledge, and knowledge allows for the higher human impulses to manifest in union with the laws of nature. When a male is born he is not capable of reproducing until he can produce sperm, at the onset of puberty. Until then he is basically infertile. A woman, on the other hand, begins her earthly life as a fetus with six to seven million eggs at twenty weeks of gestation, dropping to one to two million at birth. From then on she spends her entire life losing her eggs, lacking the ability to produce new eggs.

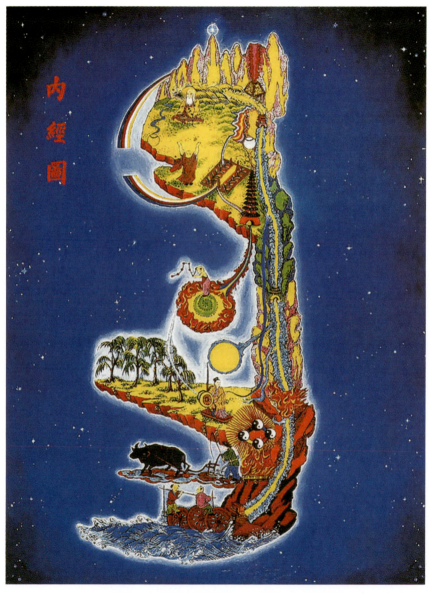

Fig. 2.1. Alchemy of Taoist Transformations

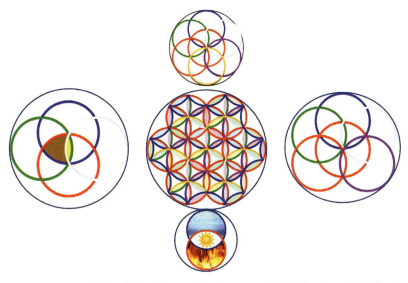

Fig. 2.2. A mandala of the Flower of Life, a symbol of the Seed of Life, the Fruit of Life, the Tree of Life, and the Egg of Life, all of which have a prominent role in explaining the creation of the universe and the creation of human life.

Men constantly replenish their sperm resources once they've been spent. Their vitality is determined by his DNA, his lifestyle, and the ecology of his environment.

All Taoist teachings refer to transformative processes: mixing, fusing, condensing, compressing, absorbing, penetrating, and multiplying. In traditional Taoist teachings, absolute mindfulness of these transformative processes provides the path to enlightenment, as does unwavering belief and trust in the help of nature, perceived as the five elements and the eight trigrams.

The human body is viewed as a microcosm that lives by the same laws of the macrocosm that is the universe. Taoist tenets are associated with the multi-orgasmic universe as an initiation in immortality. Since humans are a microcosm of the universe, the essence of human life on Earth is also multi-orgasmic, spiritual, emotional, and physiological.

And it all starts the moment when the eyes of future lovers, potential parents, meet. Taoist teachings say the act of lovemaking can result either in the loss or the acquisition of energy by the organs in the human body, so they consider sex to be an opportunity to cultivate the kind of emotional virtue that increases chi. All this depends on the physical health of the person and their emotions, all of which are imprinted on the five main organs of the human body: the heart, spleen, lungs, kidneys, and liver. These organs, in turn, have an impact on their assistants, which are functionally dependent on them: the small intestine and tongue; the

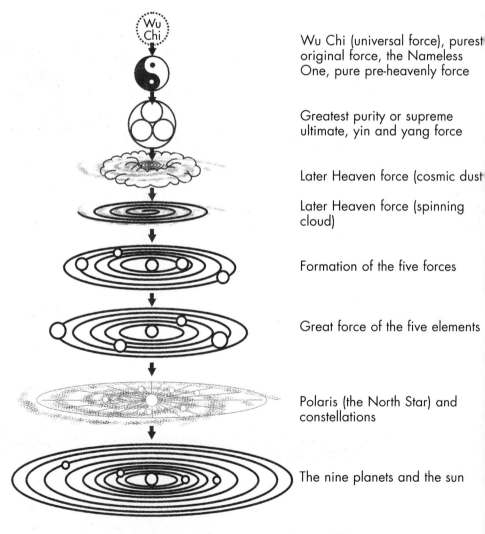

Fig. 2.3. Formation and continuing evolution of the universe

pancreas, stomach, and mouth; the large intestine and colon, skin, and bronchi; the bladder, reproductive organs, and ears; the gallbladder and the eyes. All these organs are involved in sexual arousal and orgasm, not just the sex organs. The stronger the intimacy between the lovers, the more spiritual the sex act is and the more passionate their ecstasy of love will be. It is this ecstasy that makes the orgasm rise up to the heart and fill the mind with joy, contributing to better health and longevity.

THE ALCHEMY OF LOVE

The Alchemy of Love is only present in the biorhythms of life when the man's seed is not spent spontaneously and the woman's menstrual blood is only partially poured out and partially absorbed in the blood and lymph. To achieve longevity and remain healthy, your lovemaking must always be done consciously, by learning the arts of the intimate chambers and harmonizing your feelings and emotions. These practices are not difficult to learn if you are willing to discipline your mind and expand your consciousness. In the Tao this is achieved through basic meditations: the Microcosmic Orbit, the Inner Smile, and the Six Healing Sounds. These foundational Taoist practices are excellent preparation for conscious parenthood: conception, pregnancy, childbirth, and the cultivation of the magical child. Through these transformative purifications we can create the very essence of life, the pearl of pure consciousness. With the help of these practices it is possible to conceive an immortal spiritual child who, if the intention is there, can become a beautiful physical baby. The child will be conceived in multi-orgasmic vibrations of the physical body because of the spiritual awareness of the partners. In the intimate practices described in the Tibetan and Indian Tantras, the highest culmination of sexual intercourse is achieved through ritual preparation, which creates the highest orgasm of conscious conception.

This is very different from what we find in our modern culture in which very few such sacred marriage rituals have survived. Our technological society is grounded in materialism and narcissism, which is unfortunately deeply rooted in the minds of many young people. Compassion, empathy, generosity, kindness, forgiveness—these qualities of the higher mind have all but lost their value in human interactions, creating a kind of spiritual poverty. However, if we are to consciously birth healthy, spiritually oriented children, we must practice these values. The conception of a wonderful child is directly linked to a highly spiritual orgasm, in which pure consciousness crystallizes together with the higher virtues.

The Lotus meditation is based on the balance of fire and water in our bodies. (All Chinese healing practices are based on balancing yin and yang energies.) Sometimes people struggle to conceive because of excess cold or heat in their bodies.

The Lotus Meditation

Sexual energy is connected to the kidneys and the element of water. This is a great calming and balancing practice for the entire body that both women and men can do. The heart can get overheated with worry and anxiousness, while the kidneys are often cold because of too much fear and similar blockages. This affects sexual energy, which can become cold and stagnant. This meditation restores flow and infuses the skin with a beautiful glow.

The heart, which the Tao considers a yang organ, is the origin of love. The kidneys are very yin; they are dominated by cold water energy that needs to be softened and warmed up. In naturopathic medicine, it is said that the heart and the kidneys are best friends. In this meditation we combine the sun's rays with the heat of our heart, softening it and sending it down to the kidneys, where we then imagine it sprouting lotus seeds. Through our feet—the roots of the lotus—we reach for the water, where the seeds of the lotus are found. We raise the energy of the water warmed by the rays of sun through our kidneys and direct it to the heart center, cultivating the stem, our spine. It is through the spine that the love ecstasy of the seed raises the water elixir to our heart, where the whitish-pink lotus flower blossoms. The lotus as the power of life fills our body with the colors of the rainbow, just as the flower is nourished through its stem as it gets ready to produce seeds.

Knowing Your Own Sexuality 33

The energy of fulfillment rises through our liver and our spleen, and through our entire digestive system. All these organs are lotus leaves consuming chi, the pranic energy of prosperity, furthering the continuation of life. This meditation opens the channels within and along the spine, liberating the fasciae in the organs and muscles. It is usually practiced together with the Six Healing Sounds meditation found in chapter 4, either during the day or in the evening. As an option, you can meditate by not only visualizing your own organs but also the organs of your future baby. Healing practices such as this help couples balance the emotional, physical, and spiritual bodies to strengthen their hormonal health and magnify the love in their hearts and their desire.

1. Sit on the edge of a chair. Put your feet on the floor and feel connected to the earth. Take a few deep, relaxing breaths. Smile into your body.
2. Imagine your heart as a beautiful lotus flower absorbing the energy of the sun. Feel nice and warm in your heart. Smile into your heart.

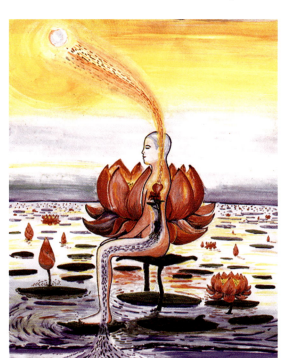

Fig. 2.4. The Lotus meditation

34   Knowing Your Own Sexuality

3. Imagine your kidneys as the bulbous roots of the lotus flower floating in cool, clear water. Smile into your kidneys.
4. Imagine your feet are the roots of the lotus flower growing deep into the muddy earth.
5. Smile into your heart and inhale. Exhale with the heart's sound, haw-w-w-w-w-w, down into your kidneys. Feel warm heart energy flowing into your kidneys, warming them up.
6. Inhale from your kidneys and exhale all the way down to the earth through your "roots."
7. Inhale from your feet up, exhaling into your kidneys.
8. Inhale from your kidneys and exhale with the kidney's sound, choo-oo-oo-oo, all the way into the heart. Feel cool, watery energy flowing into the heart, cooling it down.
9. Repeat this pattern at least 9 times, feeling your heart and kidneys balancing their energy.

Fill yourself with positive intentions by listening to spiritual music and engaging in creative activities, and you will increase your virtue and become happier—this is what the Universal Healing Tao teaches us. We come out of childhood and develop as adults so that we can continue life and increase our virtue. Failure to comply with the creative aspects of love and disharmony in our relationships can lead to miscarriage or to the baby leaving before or at the time of birth. Modern society values what it considers pragmatic interventions in preparation for conception and childbirth more than it trusts the importance of developing an inner state of peace and harmony by living according to moral and ethical standards.

BALANCING THE ELEMENTS AND ORGANS

Behavioral matrices change as a result of an increase in hormones in a woman's body, and these are transmitted to a man during the exchange of ejaculatory fluids—his "Dragon Tears" and her "Moisture of Joy," with a small amount of sperm in his fluid gathered after a series of delays to prolong the pleasure. A woman's satisfaction, in which the male seed is washed with the woman's three waters flowing out of her yoni, is extremely important for healthy conception to occur.

Since ancient times, Chinese culture has considered the highest manifestation of enlightenment to be the divine Kuan Yin, who pours her beneficial waters on humanity. Similarly, in the Thai tradition, respect for the feminine is symbolized by a beautiful young woman who has cleansing water flowing from her head, down her long hair, and into the world of humans.

Washing, cleansing, blessing, and healing with water are an important part of many spiritual traditions, both ancient and modern. Fire is required to get passion boiling, which brings the evaporating water up, crystallizing it into the immortality of the three states. Life on Earth continues in new manifestations of the elements. Until recently, no one suspected that the ability of liquid sperm to freeze allows you to preserve not only the physical substance of the sperm and egg, but also the genetic code embedded in its chromosomal memory. But what about the soul, you may ask? Perhaps it is shaped by its willingness to choose and call forth its parents.

The Inner Smile meditation is a foundational practice of the Universal Healing Tao. It focuses on balancing the energies associated with each organ, clearing any negative energy held there and amplifying the positive energies, or virtues, of each organ.

- The **heart** and **small intestine** have the positive energies of the fire element, which are love, joy, and happiness. The negative energies are hatred, cruelty, judgment, impatience, and rage.
- The **spleen**, **pancreas**, and **stomach** have the positive energies of the earth element, which are trust, faith, and confidence. The negative energies are mistrust, anxiety, worry, and self-doubt.
- The **lungs** and **large intestine** have the positive energies of the metal element, which are courage and righteousness. The negative energies are grief, depression, and sadness.

- The **kidneys** and **bladder** have the positive energies of the water element, which are calmness, tranquility, and gentleness. The negative energies are fear and stress.
- The **liver** and **gallbladder** have the positive energy of the wood element, which is generosity and kindness. The negative energies are greed, jealousy, and anger.

The Inner Smile

1. Take a deep breath, smile, look into your heart, and become aware of the fire element there. As you smile into your heart, spiral your eyes around your heart, gathering up all the excess heat. Exhale with the heart's sound, haw-w-w-w-w-w, to release excess heat from the heart. The fire element is connected to the heart and small intestine. It is connected to the positive emotions of love, joy, and happiness, as well as to the negative emotions of hatred, cruelty, judgment, impatience, and rage.
2. Become aware of the water element and your kidneys. This is connected to the positive states of calmness, gentleness, and tranquility, and to the negative emotion of fear, which is often caused by trauma or shock. To release excess water energy from the kidneys, use the kidney's sound: choo-oo-oo-oo. Also, moving cooler, calming energy from your kidneys to your heart with the kidney's sound: choo-oo-oo-oo, and moving heat from your heart to your kidneys with the heart's sound, haw-w-w-w-w-w, will balance your energy.
3. When you feel your heart is clean and clear and your kidneys are warm and calm, bring your awareness to your crown and third eye. Look through your third eye out into the universe. Then look into your heart and find the frequency of unconditional love there. Inhale the love in your heart and exhale that love out into the universe. Imagine that frequency of love being sent to galaxies far away. Become aware of the unconditional love that permeates the universe. Inhale unconditional love energy through your third eye into your heart. As you inhale universal unconditional love into your

Knowing Your Own Sexuality 37

heart, feel it increasing. Keep smiling into your heart and let the love energy increase even more. Then inhale love from your heart and exhale it through your third eye back out into the universe. Inhale unconditional love from the universe and exhale it into your heart. Feel your heart being balanced by unconditional love.

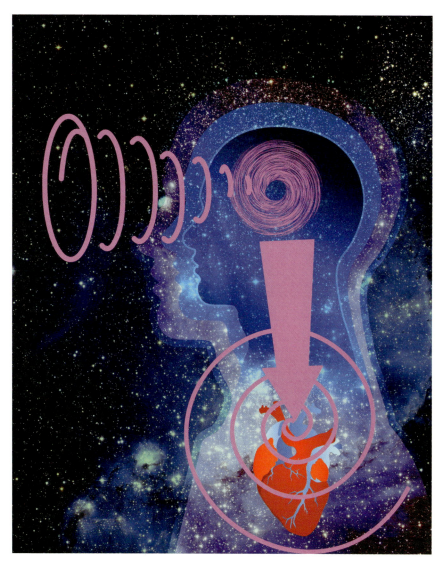

Fig. 2.5. The heart can be used to channel the unconditional love of the universe to your organs and then back again to the universe.

4. Smile into your spleen and guide unconditional love from your heart into your spleen, pancreas, and stomach. Keep smiling into your spleen and feel it being balanced. Return to your heart.

5. Smile into your lungs and guide universal unconditional love from your heart into your lungs. Keep smiling into your lungs and feel them returning to balance. Return to your heart.

6. Smile into your kidneys and guide universal unconditional love from your heart into your kidneys. Feel your kidneys returning to balance. Return to your heart.

7. Smile into your liver and guide unconditional love from your heart into your liver. Feel your liver returning to balance. Return to your heart.

8. Keep going back to your heart and replenishing the unconditional love flowing to and from the universe. Go through all your organs like this 9 times until they all are in balance.

CULTIVATING IMMORTALITY

The amazing ability of the human body to regenerate itself is not so perfected that it can live forever. Each stress we endure contributes to the death of our vital stem cells and subsequent aging.[1] The theories and practices of the Universal Healing Tao teach us how we can overcome the process of aging and significantly prolong our lives. The secret of these transformative and balancing practices lies in the purification of our consciousness, combined with absorbing the Elixir of Immortality—which happens due to the mixture of female and male secretions at the time of the highest arousal and orgasm. This is when the door to the intimate chambers is ready to be opened! You only need pick the right key to the woman's womb. That key is sexual arousal, along with the preservation and absorption of the male seed washed by amrita and the absorption of parts of menstrual blood and high-calorie colostrum intended for the formation of the embryo.

There is no emphasis on reincarnation in the Tao. The main idea is that we live long lives in health and wisdom. The path to enlightenment does not lie in limitations, but in cultivating awareness and disciplining our mind and body.

For those who embark on the path of human partnership and procreation, there's an invaluable exercise that will stimulate one's life resources. It's called the Smiling Deer. The sacred traditional form of this meditation is very simple, but it calls for the practitioner's purity of intention and a precise definition of the desired goal. The Smiling Deer meditation is the quintessential result of humans' observation of the animal world and the natural phenomena around us. In many Eastern traditions and in China, the deer is considered a mystical animal, as the speed of its movement is beyond human comprehension. In times past it happened quite often that people would report seeing the very same animal in completely different parts of the forest. They couldn't help but wonder how a deer could develop such extraordinary speed—what force was driving it? The secret lay in the sexual energy of the animal. Accelerating the vibrations of the deer's eggs or sperm by repeatedly moving the strong muscles in its triangular tail transformed its sexual arousal into speed. This is in effect the same concentrated directivity of movement of energy that takes place in the Microcosmic Orbit, described later in this chapter, with its accelerations and decelerations, whose sole purpose is powering the process of transformative creation.

The Smiling Deer

The Smiling Deer meditation has never been published before in its comprehensive and complete form. It was traditionally passed on as a priceless gift from teacher to respectful student, one who has excelled in the studies and who keeps the moral principle of "do no harm" in thoughts, words, or deeds. Taoist meditations can only reach their full power through daily practice. This mystically wonderful meditation, combined with the strong character of the practitioner and his or her unwavering intent, assists in a highly spiritual conception and resolves any problematic situations related to the quality of eggs and sperm. Many women were able to conceive their long-awaited child by practicing the Smiling Deer daily.

40   *Knowing Your Own Sexuality*

The Smiling Deer comes from the time of the legendary Yellow Emperor (ca. 2704–2696 BCE), the patron saint of Taoism. It is believed that thanks to such training of the Healing Tao, the reign of the Yellow Emperor was long and wise, and China at that time gained the status of the strongest state. The Smiling Deer is carried out with the use of massage, which affects not only the libido, but also the lymphatic and endocrine systems. It stabilizes blood circulation and regulates the engagement of the energy centers, or chakras. This technique is based on the excitation of the basic force of chi—its circulation, multiplication, and preservation in the main life center and the body's biobattery, the lower tan tien. Only in the belly can you keep the love energy of the heart and the sexual arousal of the reproductive organs. If you practice the love mysteries of Taoism, then love will not be destroyed by one's mundane, day-to-day obligations, and children will continue to be conceived, nurtured, and born in the loving union of their parents.

The prelude to this practice is the Inner Smile, which is not only directed at all the organs, meridians, bones, brain, lymphatic system, blood, and reproductive systems, but also awakens the intention behind the Smiling Deer practice.

1. The correct form for the performance of the ritual is very important: a straight back. Sit on the edge of the chair, legs shoulder-width apart, knees bent at a 90-degree angle. The toes are spread, rooting the foot to the ground through the ball of the foot below the toes and between two soft pads.
2. At first, the hands are either resting on the knees or facing whichever organ you are focusing on. It is important to free your head from any thoughts and turn your consciousness to the lower tan tien.
3. Then, the palms of the hands are turned up toward the sky, with their healing lights and colors of the rainbow.
4. Now, turning the centers of both palms toward your nipples (both woman and men can do this practice) and feeling the contact, cover your breasts with the palms of your hands and massage, rotating 36 times clockwise and 36 counterclockwise. Visually connect the feel-

ing of arousal with your ovaries or prostate gland as you change the direction of the rotation.

5. Warm the hands by rubbing them together. Carry hot sexual energy to the kidneys by briskly rubbing them, increasing sexual arousal in them as well as in the bladder, which crystallizes the internal waters.

6. Slide your hands down to heat your ligaments in the groin area of the upper part of the legs and between the legs. The ligaments and fasciae will relax, elasticized by the warmth.

7. For men, cover the testicles and massage them with your thumbs in a circular motion—36 times both clockwise and counterclockwise (or 81 times in case of disease). For women, warm up the ovaries and uterus using circular movements of the hands, touching the clitoris.

8. When the arousal is tangible, clench the palms of your hands into fists, place them on your knees, flex your toes, contract your ocular muscles by letting your eyes roll back into your head, and direct your gaze inside and up.

9. Through 9 breathing cycles, push your sexual energy through the channels of your spine to the very top of your head.

10. Flex your sex muscles and tighten up your anus and perineum. We fuel the state of arousal by the power of our glands, brain, and intention. Raise this sensation to your crown chakra and then let it fall down through the roof of your mouth and your tongue. The sweet sensation, dripping like honey, will descend through the organs to the Hui Yin point in your crotch, located at the very root of the torso, at the center of the pelvic floor, a half inch in front of the anus. The cascading sensation is enriched with the energy of sperm and eggs, as well as with the "crystallized living water" of the bladder. This orbit is performed in 9 full rotations; on the tenth, capture the energy by passing it down through the front channel, packing virtuous intent in the lower tan tien.

11. Mix the accumulated chi with the virtues, or positive qualities, of the organs and release those virtues to be implemented by each of the organs.

We offer this training not only for the purpose of preparing for procreation but also to help you fulfill your purpose in this world. Students of the Tao give this practice a 100 percent success rate, provided the future parents also do the daily physical practices of Chi Kung and Tai Chi, along with the basic meditations of the Universal Healing Tao. The basics of Healing Love are very important. The future parents must do the prescribed breath work, develop healthy nutrition, include water blessings, and purify their thoughts and words. That is how they ultimately change their DNA. Taoism maintains that it is entirely natural for a psychologically healthy person to spontaneously multiply their stem cells and modify the quality of their physical systems and spiritual body in a positive way.

Learning the notes of love through arousal and orgasm as transformative practices for accumulating and not wasting the life force is the idea behind the Universal Healing Tao. Forming the immortal energetic fetus is the basis for conceiving a wonderful child in all respects—a concept that can be credited to American author and child development expert Joseph Chilton Pearce (1926–2016), who wrote

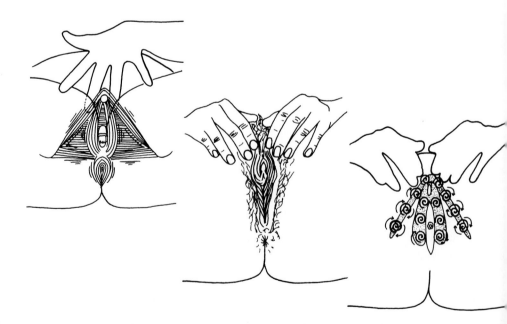

Fig. 2.6. Massaging the genitals

twelve books, including *Magical Child* and *Magical Child Matures*. These books argue that there's an impact on the quality of the gradual formation of the embryo and its bonding with its parents, especially the mother, in the womb while the child grows and develops.

INTEGRATING MICROCOSM WITH MACROCOSM

We humans came into this world purely for love, which is why the cosmos, driven by love's orgasmic energy, needs us. Yin and yang, as positive and negative impulses, create new galaxies as a result of the attraction and penetration of negatively and positively charged particles. A huge number of negatively charged particles, repelled at quite a distance from positive ones, are then attracted back to them at a very high speed, which creates a push of penetration with both quantitative and qualitative energy. Black holes are formed, and their vibrations give birth to new galaxies. In the same way the human microcosm similarly gives birth to new life by activating the energy of the eggs and the sperm, the yin and the yang. The strength and health of the stem cells, which multiply in orgasm, depend on the quality of love expressed in the orgasmic vibrations. This is the principle on which the Microcosmic Orbit meditation is based. The result leads to the creation of the bright pearl, the forerunner of the birth of the Immortal Fetus.

Taoist masters say there are two major energy highways that together follow a path around the body; they call this the Microcosmic Orbit. The first channel is the Yang Channel, which is the Governor Channel. It starts at the perineum, flows through the tailbone, inside the sacrum, up the spinal cord under the skin, under the skull to the crown, and then down the skull to the third eye and mid-eyebrow, through the sinuses, to the hard palate. The other channel is the Yin Channel, which is also called the Functional or Conception Channel. It starts at the perineum, goes up under the skin, following the midline through the navel, solar plexus, heart center, throat center, to the lower jaw. The two channels become one closed circuit, or orbit, when the tongue is lifted and pressed to the upper palate. Using mind, eye, and heart power, we can direct the flow of energy through this orbit, which distributes chi from the major energy centers throughout the body, preventing excesses and blockages.

The main points of the Microcosmic Orbit are:

1. **Navel:** The Microcosmic Orbit starts and ends at the navel center, located 1.5 inches below the navel. The navel is our first connection to the outside world from which we received nutrition and oxygen while in the womb. This area retains its energetic significance throughout life. The navel is the point for centering and connection to all the organs. It is also the entrance to the lower tan tien cauldron, which is the place where we gather, transform, and store energy.

2. **Sexual center:** In men this is called the Sperm Palace, which starts at the base of the penis. In women it's called the Ovary Palace, which is located above the pubic bone. To find the Ovary Palace, place your thumbs on your navel and make the index fingers come together below. Where two index fingers meet is the location of the Ovary Palace. The area where the pinkie fingers naturally touch is where ovaries are located. Sexual energy is the only energy that can be transformed into the life force and multiplied. When this energy is not used for procreation, it is easily lost through excessive sexual activity.

3. **Perineum, or the Gate of Life and Death:** Located between the anus and the sexual organ, the perineum is a very important point connected to the pelvic floor. If the pelvic floor is weak, this point is where the life force may leak out. If the pelvic floor is strong, a person can use the muscle of the pelvic floor to draw energy into the body.

4. **Sacrum:** In the Microcosmic Orbit there are two points connected to the sacrum, the tailbone and the sacrum itself. It's easier to just focus on the sacrum and let the energy flow from the perineum up the tailbone and up the sacrum. The sacrum is considered a pump that moves spinal fluid to the brain. Moving

the base of the spine and using the mind to move energy up the spine helps keep the brain young and vibrant.

5. **Kidney center, or the Door of Life:** This center is located on the spine opposite the navel and corresponds to the lumbar vertebrae 2 and 3 (L2 and L3). This point is connected to our prenatal energy, which is the original force. When people live in stress and fear they deplete this energy, and this weakens the entire body. The kidney's energy can be replenished with the Inner Smile meditation.

6. **Adrenal gland center:** The adrenal gland center is located on the spine at thoracic vertebra 11 (T11), opposite the solar plexus center. This center is controlled by the adrenal glands and is very sensitive to stress.

7. **Center opposite the heart:** This center is located on the spine, at thoracic 11, opposite the heart center. This center is closely connected to the heart and can contribute to creating the heart's radiance.

8. **Point opposite the throat:** This point is easy to find by locating the big protruding vertebra at the base of the neck, which is cervical vertebra 7 (C7). This point connects energy from the body to energy in the higher energy centers in the brain.

9. **Small brain point, or Jade Pillow:** This point is located above the last cervical vertebra at the base of the skull. It is connected to breathing, and when it is open it is believed that it helps us receive insights from the universe. This point is connected to the crown and third eye and stores yin energy.

10. **Crown and Crystal Palace:** The crown point is located at the top of the head. To find this point, draw a line connecting the tips of the ears and going through the highest point of the head, and another line starting from the point between the two eyebrows all the way up to the base of the skull. This is an important energy point of connection to the forces of the universe.

11. **Mid-eyebrow point and third eye:** The mid-eyebrow point is energetically connected to the pituitary gland, while the third eye

point in the middle of the forehead is connected to the pineal gland. These two points can be used together as one center. The collective location of the important endocrine glands in the brain corresponds to the Crystal Palace in the middle of the brain. These points enable connection to higher wisdom and universal light.

12. **Heavenly Pool:** This is the point located on the roof of the mouth. When you place the tip of your tongue there, the two channels, yin and yang, become one orbit. There are three positions of the tongue: the wind position, located behind the front teeth, is the easiest position to start with; the fire position, which connects to the heart energy, is located further back on the palate; and the water position at the back.

13. **Throat point:** This point is in the V-shaped space between the two collarbones. The throat point is connected to speech and communication. In Taoist philosophy, the tongue is a sense organ of the heart, and the throat point serves as an important energy bridge between the two.

14. **Heart center:** The heart energy center on the Microcosmic Orbit is located on a direct line between the navel and the throat center, one inch above the tip of the sternum. The heart center can be opened with love, joy, and happiness. For women, the heart center is very important because according to the Tao, a woman's heart center has to be open in order for her sexual energy to flow without blockages.

15. **Solar plexus center:** The solar plexus center is located halfway between the heart center and the navel. It is connected to the spleen, pancreas, stomach, and liver. A strong solar plexus deters negative emotions and radiates a strong aura, like a little sun.

16. **Point under the knees:** This point can store additional spiritual energy.

17. **Bubbling Spring point:** This point is located on the balls of both feet, in the soft spot or depression there. This point can draw in the earth force and is important for practicing grounding and stability.

18. **Big toe:** This point is on the lateral side of each big toe, and it helps balance spiritual energy.
19. **Kneecap:** This point is in the middle of the upper portion of both knees. It helps refine earth energy as it goes up the legs.

 ## The Microcosmic Orbit

The Microcosmic Orbit starts and ends at the navel. It unites you as an integrated whole, with mind, body, and spirit flowing together, elevating your energy. Before you begin, review all 19 points of the Microcosmic Orbit above, and locate them on your body. Tap them if they are easy to access and breathe into the points that are more difficult to reach. To move energy, use your smile, your eyes, and your mind to guide chi. The more you learn to focus inwardly and the more you learn to smile and relax, the more you will feel how real chi moves through your body, bringing light and life to all the organs and cells.

1. Begin at your navel and move your energy down to your perineum and up to your Door of Life, located on your spine directly across from your navel. Then smile into your adrenal gland center, the point on your spine across from your solar plexus, and imagine pulling the energy up your spine to your adrenal gland center. Exhale, relax, and smile.
2. Smile into the area on your spine across from your heart center. This is the Wing point. Inhale and pull the energy up to this point. Exhale, smile, and relax.
3. Gently tap the point opposite the throat, on the protruding neck vertebrae (C7). Smile into your C7. Inhale and pull energy up to this point. Exhale, smile, and relax.
4. Gently tap your Jade Pillow at the base of your skull and smile into it. Pull energy up into your Jade Pillow.
5. Smile into your crown and put your tongue on the roof of your mouth. There are three locations on the roof of your mouth—front (behind the teeth), middle, and back. Explore which one allows

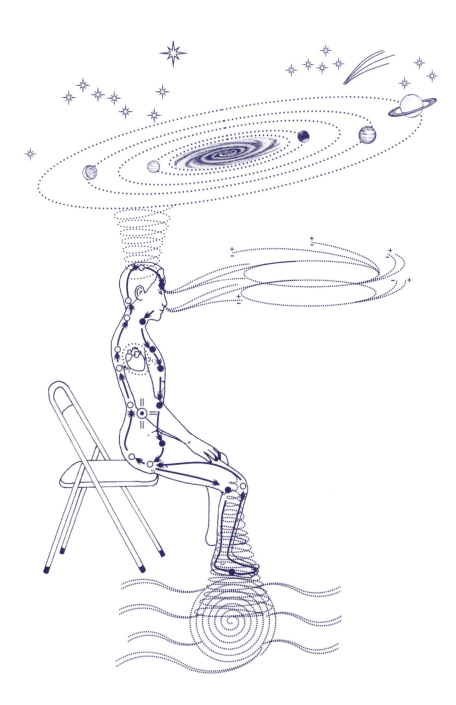

Fig. 2.7. The Microcosmic Orbit

for a more noticeable energy flow. Later you can try alternating between them. Guide chi up to your crown.
6. Smile down into your third eye and into your physical eyes. Imagine your eyes becoming cooler and more relaxed. Then smile and let chi flow down through your sinuses to the roof of your mouth, to your tongue, throat, heart center, and solar plexus, and finally to your navel. Keep the energy moving through this orbit, directing it with your attention and focus. Remember to smile and relax.
7. When you're done, collect chi in your navel by massaging your belly around the outside of your navel (not in the navel) 24 times counterclockwise, expanding the spiral. Then massage in the opposite direction, 36 times, concentrating energy in the navel. Imagine there is a small cauldron in your navel where you collect energy.
8. When you become more familiar with moving the orbit through your body, you can expand it from your perineum to the soles of your feet, and then up your legs and into your perineum again. The orbit flows in a figure-eight pattern, so when you reach the perineum, moving from the navel, you continue from the perineum down the back of your thighs to the points under your knees and down to the Bubbling Spring, and then to your big toe point and up the front of your legs to your kneecap point and then back to your perineum, to continue up your tailbone and up your spine.

Eventually all you will need to do is to think about your orbit and send energy flowing, and it will flow like a river, nourishing your whole body. The Microcosmic Orbit eventually becomes the Macrocosmic Orbit, where you let the figure-eight pattern continue to include the sun, the moon, and the planets, as well as the earth. This creates an expansive, radiant feeling and refines your energy.

 ## The Microcosmic Orbit for Partners

In this version of the Microcosmic Orbit, you are exchanging energies with your partner, which creates a synergy.

1. To open the orbital channels penetrating the spine and passing alongside it, we recommend that a couple work together in this exercise. One of the partners sits on a chair, feet resting flat on the floor, legs open, chin tucked, and the neck freely stretched. The palms are open and rest on the knees, eyes closed.
2. The assistant stands on the left side of the chair and with the hands aligning the field of peace and harmony. Both practitioners should concentrate on the area between the eyebrows and relax the mind.
3. The assistant's left hand rests opposite the tan tien. The right hand feels the Door of Life directly across from the navel on the spine. Soft rotational movements of the palms on that area help to open deeper and more subtle sensations.
4. The hands of the assistant then rise to the top of the head and then fall to the tailbone.
5. The assistant's right hand starts to move in tapping motions at the tailbone, while the left hand slides up along the front downward

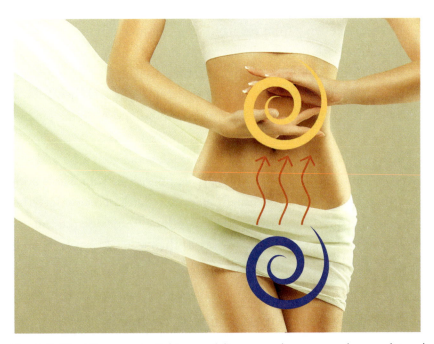

Fig. 2.8. The Microcosmic Orbit can deliver sexual energy and unconditional love to all the organs and cells of the body.

Knowing Your Own Sexuality **51**

channel. Each area is tapped on with three fingers pinched together to resemble a bird's beak.

6. In unison, while the assistant is tapping around the tailbone area, both participants should flex their perineal region on an inhalation and push the energy higher to the sacrum and above T11, T10, then to the 5 and 4 thoracic vertebrae (opposite the heart center).

7. The assistant then moves to the area of the convex cervical vertebra, the protruding point at the base of the neck, and from there the "beak" is directed to the Jade Pillow, the point above the last cervical vertebra at the base of the skull.

8. It is important to feel the vibration with the glands located at this level in the head—the hypothalamus, pituitary, epiphysis, and cerebellum. The crown of the head is an important location where chi twists into a spiral, going upward in one direction and in the opposite direction twisting down; then going through the middle of the eye to the roof of the mouth.

9. Press your tongue against the upper palate and then down to the center of your throat, then to the thymus, softly through the heart, through the solar plexus, to the tan tien, where a portion of the energy is stored and a part is channeled through the sex organs of the groin region to the Hui Yin, located at the very root of the torso, at the center of the pelvic floor, a half inch in front of the anus.

10. The Hui Yin is where we twist and untwist the sensation of power in a spiral, with the purpose of holding and saving the energy. Continue to move it up and down in an elliptical shape. Don't forget to breathe in unison with compression of the sex muscles.

11. Move the orbit around no less than 3 times, and on the fourth round both partners should capture it and pack the chi strongly in the life center, located two fingers below the navel.

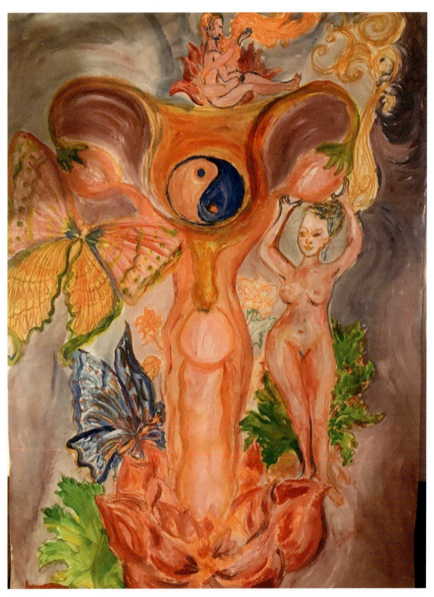

Illustration by Marina Dadasheva-Drown

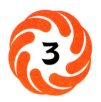

3
The Alchemy of Conception

What is nature guided by when it brings two people together as partners? Let's not consider the whole computer dating thing; instead, let's consider traditional matchmaking done by the parents, who would choose a groom for the bride or vice versa. In the past (and occasionally even now), this was a way of controlling young people or a practical way to grow the population of healthy children. In India, in stable and respected families, marriages were sometimes arranged for kids even while they were still in infancy. Sometimes the children in these arranged marriages grew up together, so there was a feeling of kinship and a deep affection between them that eventually grew into sexual attraction and the social pressure to create a family. In more or less equal marriages, where no partner depended on the other financially, there usually was harmony—respect for social and religious traditions, the elders, and for each other. The wealth of the family was determined by well-raised children and their later life choices.

Times have indeed changed, but the ancient traditions of the Kama Sutra and the Vedic and Taoist heritage of the art of love continues to this day in the teachings of the Universal Healing Tao. In families that cultivate the notes of love, a virtual symphony is created that can be heard and understood by the children in such fortunate circumstances.

54   The Alchemy of Conception

In ancient Taoist tradition, rituals and deeply intimate ceremonies conducted at the moment of conception were fundamental to the further bonding of a couple. Chastity and knowledge of the mysteries of intercourse were aligned with the phases of the lunar cycle and were highly valued. Awareness and skill in lovemaking came from both the groom and the bride. The couple was prepared for family life by experienced mentors versed in the mysteries of the Kama Sutra and sexual Tantra. The dances and songs of these disciplines opened the gates of love.

In ancient Chinese tradition, matchmaking was very highly valued. Partners selected through matchmakers had the potential not only to create but also to ennoble their families with healthy offspring. Not so long ago, a man could have several wives, a decision that was determined by his wealth and the ability of his wife to satisfy his love appetite and bear enough children. Since the times of the Yellow Emperor and his descendants, internal martial arts were practiced in order to transform sexual creativity into health and high spirituality. This form of martial arts is a powerful and highly effective discipline where the practitioner remains relatively soft and flexible, moving like water or wind. Women, like men, trained their bodies and expanded their consciousness in such practices. To become a wife or concubine, prepubescent girls were trained in erotic dance and learned how to strengthen the elasticity of their hymen and sexual muscles by training with a jade egg (see chapter 1). The ability to arouse and be aroused, to own the art of her intimate muscles and to take care of the beauty and milkiness of her breasts, was as natural to a girl as learning to play the flute and mastering the art of making tea and preparing food. A woman was valued for her strength, skillfulness, and femininity.

Erotic massage imbued with healing properties was and still is widely practiced in almost all Asian cultures as a prelude to intimacy. To arouse the girl and bring out her natural sexual desire and her ability to experience pleasure and the ecstasy of love, the young man was obligated to open her secret gates of love by using the skills of his tongue, his fingers, and his toes, as well as his Jade Wand (his penis). The erotic massage usually included elements of the ancient art of

Karsai Nei Tsang,* a form of therapeutic massage of the sexual organs that heals injuries and relieves menstrual pain. By affecting the fasciae, muscles, and joints of the hip area, Karsai (from the inside) and Chi Nei Tsang (massage of internal organs from the outside) relax the woman and future mother and free her sexuality and her fantasies. The couple is likened to two deities creating a love that can combat human vices—Shakti and Shiva enjoying the erotica of their relationship, joining nature in their ecstasy, discovering the taste of life to the sounds of the flute and by observing nature.

Music is always present in love ceremonies, as is ecstasy and joint creativity. The ritual sharing of a drink from mouth to mouth and being fed exotic foods that symbolize the five elements and senses by your lover are typical of these kinds of rituals. There's a ritual in the White Tantra called the Five M's, or Panchamakara, which cultivates the opening of the sense of taste not through sexual ecstasy, but from tasting the five elements and sharing them with your lover. A similar practice is performed in Taoist Healing Love when lovers embrace, warm each other's kidneys, and exchange Microcosmic Orbits (see the Microcosmic Orbit for Partners in chapter 2), raising their sexual energies up their spines with the help of their breath. Having filled the mind and root glands with the elixir of chi, lovers lower it with a golden honey stream of virtues through the organs down to the point of Hui Yin, in the perineum. This area is the repository of female yin power.

The female aspect of sexuality is also inherent in a man for the balance of his individual creativity. The essence of male energy, the focus of which is the Million Dollar point (see chapter 1), is also necessary for a woman. In the ecstasy of intercourse, she receives the fluids of his male power along with its vitamins as she soaks up the Tears of the Dragon, or precum. The area of the cherished, precious, Million Dollar point is easy to determine with the help of the fingers, a small dip closer to the anus than to the scrotum. The Hui Yin point

---

*See Master Chia's book *Karsai Nei Tsang: Therapeutic Massage for the Sexual Organs* (Destiny Books, 2011).

is close to it, closer to the front of the muscle, under the testicles. The perineum has the power of muscles that can stop the flow of the seed and reserve it for transformation into the vital energy of the organs and brain. These life forces must gather together for conception to occur. The Tao teaches us to honor our age and seasonal restrictions when it comes to the delay of ejaculation and take into account the individuality of a man, including his blood type, his temperament, and his lifestyle. The woman is offered daily breast massage, kneading the area from the armpits to the nipples and applying pressure in circular motions while lightly pinching the nipples. Caressing and massaging the breasts, which arouses the nipples, labia, and clitoris, is a ritual practice that every woman should do in the morning and in the evening to prepare for conception.

THE ENERGY OF THE HEART IN SEXUALITY

For a long time science held that the emotions are controlled solely by the brain and depend on its functional state. More recently, however, as a direct result of the return of respect for the ancient traditions, this notion has changed such that it has become quite obvious that it is the heart that creates a hormonal surge and a subsequent state of arousal.

Drunvalo Melchizedek, in his book *Living in the Heart: How to Enter into the Sacred Space within the Heart*, discusses the features of the human heart. He tells us that the development of the embryo starts with the heart, not the brain. He brings up a discovery made by researchers at the HeartMath Institute that may just be the answer to scientists' question as to where the impulse that awakens and regulates the heartbeat comes from. He says the heart has a brain of its own, that it in fact contains brain cells. There are about forty thousand of these cells, so this brain of the heart is relatively small, but this is enough for the heart, confirming the validity of "thinking with the heart," in which the wisdom of the heart comes as a feeling, a knowing without question, or a familiar voice that comes from the higher self.

The Tao is neither a science nor a religion. It is a practical guide to the health of the human body, with the heart as its main power supply. If there is not enough spiritual love in it, then there is no energy for the orgasmic engagement of the kidneys and the glands involved in basic sexual energy, which contributes to feelings of happiness, desire, and the ability to procreate. This kind of love deficiency means that there aren't enough impulses of the heart—no desire to share the overwhelming abundance of emotions, excitement, and sexual vibrations, not only with your partner, but also with your child before and after birth. Ancient sources claim that the quality and duration of childbirth depend on a woman's ability to love her child. It is said that sometimes it takes at least three days to open a woman's heart. If after that time the mother's heart does not fill with compassion and love, the child's soul has the right to go to other prospective parents—or it may die in utero or choose not to incarnate.

> Let rapture be preserved at each approach to a new consciousness. A hardened heart will not ascend to the Tower. It will not give strength to the subtle body. Such a stony heart will remain within the confines of Earth. It is very important to understand the life of the heart. One should not permit it to revert to primeval stone. One should watch over the manifestations of the heart. Without it, Brotherhood cannot be built.[1]

When modern experiments with artificial fertilization of the egg outside the mother's body first began, there were many failures because the man, the center of love and sexual desire, was not directly involved in the process. If the woman helped him get the sperm herself and the man caressed his beloved and held her hand at the time of fertilization, when the sperm was deposited in the woman's womb, positive results increased many times over. Not all fertilized eggs would take root in the uterus, however, if there was not enough oxytocin, the necessary hormone of love—which happens when a woman undergoes this procedure in a sterile clinic and not in her love nest, in the arms of her beloved.

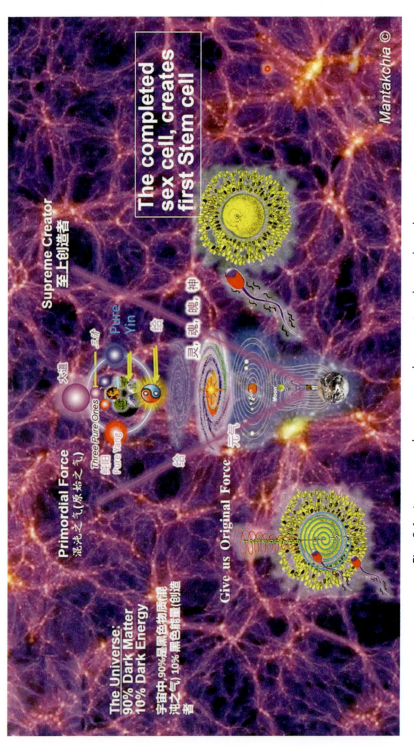

Fig. 3.1. A sperm and an egg, and conception during their division

Once conception has taken place, gentle, loving intercourse, which feeds the mother's womb with male vitamin secretions, can only help consolidate the pregnancy and does not pose any risk whatsoever. It is undeniable that conception requires appropriate energy, not just physical cells. And now it has been proven by scientists at the HeartMath Institute that compared to other organs, including the brain, the heart generates the largest and most powerful energy field. Creating this field of loving energy is absolutely necessary in order to conceive. Couples who experience issues with conception must understand the primacy of heart energy before turning to doctors and undergoing all kinds of tests that can damage the energy of love with the kind of fear and apprehension usually associated with this medical process. We base this on some thirty years of experience dealing with such situations, and the result is always positive if the couple doesn't run into ideological conflicts in this regard. Unfortunately, the medical system's narrow-mindedness and a tendency to only trust in surgical and medical interventions does not support a healthy gene pool in our modern society. Once Marina worked with a not-so-young couple who were ready for parenthood. The doctors advised them not to waste any time on spontaneous conception and directed them to IVF. They tried artificial insemination three times, and it did not work, and they eventually came to the author out of complete desperation. A calling of the souls was on the agenda! And what happened? The couple realized that they were not a good fit for each other and separated. Amazingly, each of them was able to conceive with their new partners without medical intervention.

CREATIVITY IN LOVEMAKING

The Universal Healing Tao repeatedly brings our attention to the relationship between all the major organs of the body. If the heart can "think" with the energy of love on the cellular level, then various other emotions are created and live in the other organs, too, so we can assume that they too have the cellular memory of reproduction. The

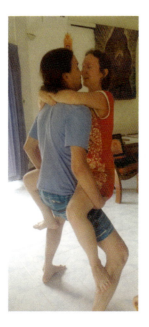

Fig. 3.2. Lovemaking pose, comfortable during pregnancy and breast-feeding

Tao assigns this function to the fasciae, which are the binding basis of each organ and the surrounding muscles. Fasciae are thin membranes of white, almost transparent color. They tense and relax, just like ligaments. In a tense state they retain tense emotions; in a relaxed state they are virtuous, calm, and joyful.

Variety in sexual positions improves a couple's bond. When a man and a woman are well-aware of the features of their physiques and the parameters of their sex organs, it is easier for them to express sexual creativity with each other. In Taoist practice we start by putting our erogenous zones on display so we can carefully study the physiology of the structure of the yoni—the clitoris, perineum, and vagina—and that of the phallus and the rest of the male anatomy; we can then penetrate into the secret parts of the beloved. This process requires patience, attention, and respect. For each couple there are always more suitable positions for achieving both pleasure and conception (or for avoiding pregnancy). The Taoist culture of lovemaking is based on our awareness and curiosity. There are also recommendations based on knowledge of the depth and strength of the vagina as well as the height of the perineum.

For a woman with a small yoni (called a *gazelle*), which corresponds with a high perineum, the upper, frontal poses are preferable as well as on the side (belly to belly), which allows for a penis of any size to reach the proximity of the cervix. If a woman has a low perineum (up to one centimeter) and a fairly deep and wide vagina (called an *elephant*), positions from the back or on the side are recommended. If the yoni is of average size (no higher than two centimeters, called the *buffalo* or *tigress*), you can enjoy poses from both the top and the bottom to vary intercourse while using your imagination and knowledge of the sutras. In this case, conception depends on the virtuosity of the partners and their level of energy.

Couples who practice Chi Kung have an opportunity to get creative in a standing position. For example, the man standing in tree position hugs the woman around the area of her kidneys, while the woman, in one strong up movement, stands on his slightly bent knees in a half squat, convenient for rocking in different directions. Her pelvis is open and ready to accept his sperm, with the idea being to conceive. The woman flexes the muscles of her sex organs and with each movement pulls the energy fluids into her uterus, filling it with the necessary hormonal secretions that constitute the Elixir of Immortality.

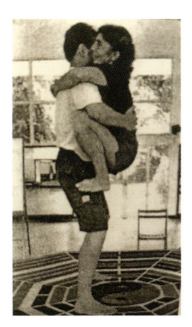

Fig. 3.3. The man standing in tree position hugs the woman around her kidneys.

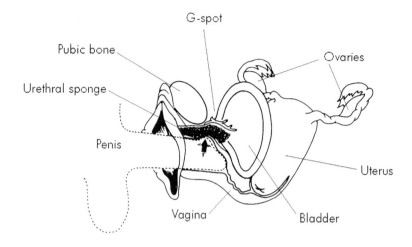

Shallow thrust massages the area of the G-spot.

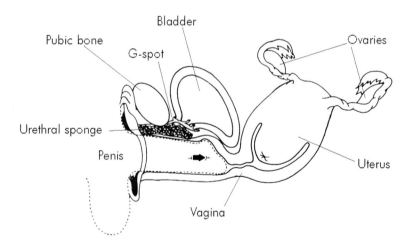

Deep thrust massages the deeper areas of the vagina, bypassing the G-spot.

Fig. 3.4. Massage of the G-spot during intercourse

In a woman's perineal region, between the anus and the pelvic diaphragm, there is another strong muscle, the urogenital diaphragm. The urethra passes through this muscle, and the body of the clitoris is attached to it on either side, which when flexed presses on the urethral sponge and the G-spot, causing the blood to flow and pushing the orgasmic momentum higher. The tension of both diaphragms prevents the leakage of sexual chi that Taoist call *Ching* through the holes of the lower body, which helps to improve the circulation of chi in the organs. By diversifying their positions in a sexual act, a couple can prevent premature ejaculation and increase the secretions for both men and women—his Tears of the Dragon (precum) and her ejaculative fluids of amrita.

If the woman does not intend to conceive, then after ejaculation she should push the energy down from her abdomen into her perineum and then pull it up to her head along her spine, using the force of the coccygeal muscle. In this case it is always good to assume a vertical position. If she wants to conceive, and so that the sperm will not pour out of her yoni before reaching an egg, she should remain in a lying-down position and allow the energy to collect in the lower part of her belly and from there to be absorbed by her cervix, uterus, and fallopian tubes. At this point the woman's intimate waters dilute the ejaculate, a process known as "the spring flows into the ocean," which happens only after his semen becomes more agile and not sticky. The process of dilution requires at least twenty minutes.

Copulation should be a highly spiritual ceremony that passes on the subconscious knowledge of love and sexuality to the newly forming human. American ethnographer and mystic of the twentieth century Carlos Castaneda reveals to us the unique views of Yaqui sorcerers. In their system of knowledge, a human is a cocoon of luminous threads, the ends of which begin and end in infinity. These are energy threads. "The only real energy we possess is a life-bestowing sexual energy," Carlos's teacher, Don Juan, tells him. It is a root force that lasts the entire life of a human being. We use it at our discretion—waste it, multiply it, or manipulate it. Human awareness begins to develop from the moment of conception. The sorcerer Genaro, a colleague of Don Juan, tells Carlos, "The nagual Julian used to say that to have sex is a matter of energy. For instance, he never had any problems having sex because he had bushels of energy. But he took one look at me and prescribed right away that my peter was just for peeing. He told me that I did not have enough energy to have sex. He said that my parents were too bored and too tired when they made me. He said that I was the result of very boring sex, *cojida aburrida*. I was born like that, bored and tired."

It seems that our entire generation neglected thinking about the mood in which to conceive children. The basic attitude of so many people today seems to be, "Why have children at all when the planet is already overpopulated?" How many generations before us did not have the knowledge to undertake inspired, conscious parenthood? How many generations to come will lack awareness of the importance of love and gratitude when it comes to sexuality? Since ancient times, both in India and in China, in the Brahmin and Taoist traditions, marital relations were built ritually; the phases of coitus were performed as a ritual, especially when it came to conception and pregnancy. From Rajbali Pandey's book *Hindu Samskaras: Socio-Religious Study of the Hindu Sacraments*, we learn about the ritual preceding the act of love. The man was likened to Heaven and the woman to Earth. The man approached his wife saying, "I am the Sky, you are the Earth. I am the melody, you are the hymn. Let us marry and have children." Pandey explains that a woman's nobility of character played quite a strong role. A man was advised not to approach his wife if "she is not worthy of praise, angry, feels bad, unkind, loves another man, or has no desire at all."

Healthy sexuality has traditionally been considered necessary for procreation and strengthening family ties. Since sexuality is the basis for the accumulation and conservation of energy in individuals and in the family, it contains information that is transmitted not only from partner to partner but also to their offspring. In the Indian foundational text on Ayurveda, the Charaka Samhita, a woman during intimacy was likened to the goddess of love, imagining herself to be in the arms of Vishnu, Shiva, or Krishna, believing that her future child will embody the features of the visualized deity.

In the Taoist "Reliable records about three levels of purity" it is said that the true yin and the true yang are the two breaths of your father and mother, and from these breaths, with the help of seed and blood, the embryo is created. Once the development of the embryo is complete, the bodily form is created. These aspects of understanding conception as the most important part of planting the seed for a gifted child are extensively discussed in the Chinese Buddhist canon *Anthology of Taoist Philosophy* (1994): "Our heart maintains an intricate dialogue with our brain, body, and world at large and selects from the hierarchy of those fields the information appropriate to our particular experience."

WATER, THE ALCHEMICAL ELEMENT

Wu Chi, the Supreme Natural Power in the universe—in Western terminology, God or Source (the primordial force)—is associated with the bedroom arts. In traditional Taoism, the highest art form is conception in water. In times past, Taoists commonly used steam rooms with wooden barrels in which partners enjoyed lovemaking. In many ancient drawings on such barrels we see frolicking children, obviously unconsciously blessing the couple to call in a new soul.

French obstetrician and childbirth specialist Michel Odent represents the new movement in obstetrics and gynecology. Odent believes that water plays a significant role when it comes to improving the human genotype, and he pays particular attention to dolphins and the interaction between the dolphin mind the human mind. During a period of reconsidering his values while studying the effects of birthing methods on subsequent life, Odent wrote the 1990 book *Water and Sexuality*, in which he acknowledges a child's personal rights as an individual, and not as a swaddled doll that needs to keep up with the scientific graphs dictating growth and recommended vaccination schedules.

Odent gives many examples of researchers who have observed dolphins ecstatically mating both above and under the water. This is how one of his informants poetically described the sight: "At the end, the pair rise high above the sea, black snouts against the sky."

With the last movement
Powerfully churning their flukes in unison for fifty feet below,
They propel themselves upwards,
Gallons of water sluicing down their sides,
They both jump clear,
Held together in midair for their massive climax.

These phenomenal animals make love many times a day, regardless of their life cycle or their age, and researchers say that water inspires sexual creativity. In these species, eroticism is not just about procreation, the same as with humans. But we are social beings, and a human's life is bound up with moral limitations, with a sense of responsibility and duty. In whales and dolphins, the nature of sexuality is quite different—it is influenced by their environment of water and a morality that is beyond our comprehension. Their sexuality is a manifestation of love for their entire intelligent species. We can say that they are bisexual, heterosexual, and homosexual, which does not affect their partnerships, performance of parental duties, and rituals associated with the birth and raising of their young. A lot of their creativity relates to life within their communities. Dolphins live in pods in which their relationships are based on helping one another, which gets expressed through their extraordinary love. It is noted that female dolphins possess a sexuality much like the total maternal love of humans. They give birth and breast-feed in the same love ecstasy. Odent refers to a Pakistani tribe that lives in the Hindu Valley, whose symbol of sexuality is a female dolphin. Nymphomaniac women, who are called *bulban* according to their legends, began their race as a result of making love to the dolphins.

In various works about what is called *freebirth* (where you choose to have a baby without the interventions of medical providers), including both oceanic and at home, questions are often asked about why dolphins come to the place where women give birth in the ocean, or why pregnant women see dolphins in their dreams. Why do dolphins circle around these newborns in the water? Why are they so interested in these babies? Maybe these smiling dolphins see these babies as their relatives and they are trying to share their knowledge of a peaceful and joyful coexistence that will change our collective future for the better. Maybe they recognize in this new generation of water-birthed children the fruits of true love and caring. It is important to note that not all parents are ready for such exceptional children—they only come to people with higher awareness who are willing to engage their creative potential.

Delfania, by Russian Romantic writer Vladimir Lermontov (1814–1841), is a very interesting novel that expresses the mission of children who are born in the water and go on to lead an aquatic lifestyle in life. These children are not afraid of water, they are friends with it. It is in their genetic code, and it is integral to their development. Perhaps this is why their consciousness is closer to that of the dolphins than those of us who came into this world by more conventional means.

In only a relatively brief period of time our planet has acquired a level of pollution that cannot sustain new life coming in. The time for purification and arousal by water has come. Most doctors and obstetricians agree that pregnancy and childbirth are best combined with swimming and rhythmic breath-holding in the water.

THE END OF SEXUALITY?

The question we are facing at this time is a radical one: will we continue the human race by means of sexual arousal and loving ecstasy, or will we reproduce by artificial insemination? In the 1960s we went through what was heralded as a "sexual revolution." Now, some sixty years later, we are on the verge of a sexual counterrevolution. The twenty-first century marks its beginning, as science attempts to bring in new life entirely without sex. Yes, this is the same generation that is saturated with commercials of a frankly pornographic nature; a generation of avid consumers of food (or artificial "food"), cosmetic surgery, and poisons such as dioxins (found in all chlorinated substances), sodium sulfates (in detergents), saxitoxins (found in water algae), and phosphates (present in meat and fish industries, used for increasing the weight of the products). This generation cannot even defend itself against the juggernaut of genetic modification and as a result is fast approaching sterility, both men and women. Most people do not want to believe, read, or hear about this. Only those who are already on the verge of despair seem to be able to take a more natural approach to life. Will we be able to rebuild human society with love and positive thoughts and actions? Will we build a new future for the people of Earth, one filled with the virtues of our cousins, the dolphins?

The state of human sexuality at this time in our history could be compared to the final stage of sexuality in a modern woman. Having passed the purity of the baby stage, a prepubescent girl encounters the very beginnings of her sexuality when she is faced with all sorts of cultural taboos in the transitional period from childhood to womanhood. These taboos remain in place during the maturation of her oocytes, the immature female gametocytes. She experiences her first hormonal surges and urgent feelings of sexual desire as a first step toward motherhood. And then there's motherhood itself, with all of the changes it brings. Then as she matures, she experiences perimenopause and the last of her remaining eggs for the creation of new life. This is followed by menopause, when she can no longer reproduce—the current state of planetary sexuality.

Can we stop the biological clock that dictates our eventual decay? The answer, of course, is a resounding no; after all, the river does not flow backward. However, it is possible to slow down aging, activate the libido, experience sexual desire in sensual contact with a partner, and make intimate discoveries and intelligent use of the precious gifts of nature for as long as we are alive.

In the past, before the Church's patriarchs began regulating human sexuality through any number of moral restrictions, people celebrated all kinds of sexual bacchanalias and ritual festivals of fertility that coincided with the natural elements and the movements of the planets. People would sanctify sexuality, raise their libido, and choose a partner for procreation during these kinds of rites. The pagan holidays deified the solar energy that nourishes the Earth and honored Earth's waters for their life-giving force. These distant ancestors lived in harmony with nature and learned from it.

When the Church stepped in to control human behavior, this led to ruthless restrictions on women as sexual beings, while male adultery was tacitly condoned (even among priests and monks). This has basically continued up to the present, with few exceptions. Modern rap music, strip bars, violent video games, and the pervasiveness of alcohol and drugs can hardly have a positive effect on the libido and one's sexual identity. Being satiated with these kinds of stimulations never created upliftment of either the mind or the body. Sexual de-energization leads to infantilism and indifference toward even the idea of healthy sex, and as a consequence, mental instability and resentment arises toward those who have managed to maintain a healthy sense of their sexuality and have not wasted their vital life force.

The founding in 2001 of an organization called the Asexual Visibility and Education Network (AVEN) to promote "asexuality [as] an intrinsic part of who we are, just like other sexual orientations" expresses current trends in human sexuality. On the heels of these harmless asexuals come the more aggressive "antisexual" movement, which expresses opposition or overt hostility toward sexual behavior and sexuality in general, and whose adherents seek to impose their insane ideas on the younger generations. Isn't it better to go back to our traditional human roots, when we considered sex and procreation to be our wealth and heritage?

A TANTRIC RITUAL DESCRIBED

One of the simplest ways of realizing your sensuality is to share the intimacy of your body—your erogenous zones and your orgasm—with your partner. This and every other tantric sex ritual is aimed at discovering your sexual divinity and affirming certain higher qualities necessary in a love partnership, such as trust, patience, and acceptance.

70   The Alchemy of Conception

Let's take a look at a typical tantric ritual:

The man and woman begin by uniting their heart energies through gentle, intimate touching, taking a vow of silence for the duration of the sexual sacrament. While dancing to a gentle melody of love, the woman undresses while the man plays an instrument and takes in her beauty. Prior to that, clothing worn by the lovers has already been coordinated with the colors of love to emphasize the beauty of the nudity that's about to follow. The woman, now fully undressed, entrusts her lover with removing her jewelry while she starts playing the flute with her eyes closed (nowadays it is completely acceptable to use recordings of erotic music). Then the man undresses, his eyes closed, as he hums a mantra. He slowly strips, gradually revealing his naked body.

Once all of his clothes and jewelry are removed, they perform a ritual embrace, and the woman takes her beloved's hand and ushers him to the bathroom, carrying a lighted candle and incense. Using a stream of water or pouring water from her hands, she washes the man with very erotic touches, as the man continues to keep their vow of silence, eyes closed, as he resists responding to her caresses. A towel is used not to rub him, but to gently wrap around him, absorbing moisture. Then the couple trades places, and the woman closes her eyes in silence. Her partner washes her entire body with water, even her intimate parts, all the way down to her toes. After soaking up the moisture of her skin with a towel, the man covers the lower part of his body with a pareo and leads the naked woman to a bed of pillows. Drowning in these pillows, she sits down and opens her legs just slightly to reveal her flower. Her lover sits opposite her at arm's length to avoid any possibility of contact and premature arousal. Candles are lit and music is played as the aroma of incense wafts through the room. With her eyes closed, the woman fills her hands with love energy then opens the palms of her hands, uttering the *Om Adi Om* mantra of Kundalini Yoga. Then she begins to gift the intimacy of her erogenous zones. First, her hands stroke her hair and then she massages her ears with the soft penetration of her index fingers, followed by her eyes, eyebrows, eyelashes, nostrils, lips, gums, tongue, palate, and teeth, touching each cell of her sanctuary with her palms and the backs of her hands. Then she inserts her fingers into her secret cave and prayerfully accepts the smell and taste of herself. After chanting the mantra, she caresses her neck, shoulders, and breasts, moistening her fingers with saliva and the smell and the taste of her most intimate waters.

Then the worship of the divine essence of motherhood takes place as she touches the erogenous zones of her abdomen, inner thighs, and legs, followed by a prayerful tasting of the healing waters as she touches her yoni. Massage of the yoni can be performed with oil or with saliva. Everything is done in a slow rhythm to softly open the main erogenous zones: the anus, perineum, vagina, and its sacred gates. Feeling the approach of orgasm as she contracts her muscles and rhythmically breathes, she raises this energy to her heart. In anticipation of the second wave of pleasure, she uses all her arousal skills to bring herself to ecstasy several times, tasting the waters of joy, and only with the final orgasm does she allow it to flow to her sex organs, filling them with the elixir of amrita that is her yoni juice, whose taste is like that of ambrosia. Her partner hugs her as he takes off his pareo and ties it around her hips.

Now it's his turn to gift her with his sexuality and open to the mystery of the male orgasm. Inspired by the woman's demonstrations of love, he too creates a symphony of his eroticism, revealing the intimacy of each part of his male divine power. He devotes this part of the ritual to his priestess of love, revealing the secrets of his sexuality to her. He uses his saliva when touching her nipples and gently massages her navel, asserting his connection with her fecundity.

His groin area can be gently moisturized with oils as he massages his testicles and nifty rod, as well as his anus and the perineum. A man should not rush through this but should rather show respect for his own masculinity. Having nearly brought himself to the critical point, he raises the energy further by breathing and flexing his muscles to move the energy up to his heart and then to his head, and then, spreading his pending orgasm throughout his body like a lotus flower, he returns to his sacred area and experiments with sensations and breathing. Having

72 The Alchemy of Conception

steadily worked up to this point, the man now pours out his elixir mixed with his Dragon Tears, enjoying the smell and taste.

All of this takes place as the couple chants mantra, their eyes closed. The man hugs his beloved, and they perform the closing ritual of the five Ms,* opening to the taste of the five elements and calling them to their side if the couple intends to conceive.

It is not recommended to have any physical contact an hour before the sexual ritual and not to engage in sexual intercourse for twelve hours afterward. This increases desire and cultivates patience. You can, however, perform the ritual of Opening the Lotus as a couple. The couple confesses to each other their intention to cultivate love in this lotus ritual. The man sits on a chair or on a round ottoman in the garden and invites the woman to sit in his lap in a cross-legged lotus position, hugging him with her legs as she touches the soles of her feet together and with her hands warms the area of his kidneys and adrenal glands, as her partner gives her the same warmth.

After whispering their intention to conceive into each other's ears, the couple, united by breath, penetrate the lotus's world by visualizing the man directing his lotus seed into her fertile soil. Smiling at their organs, they cultivate the stem and leaves of the lotus, filling their organs with virtues and visualizing the growth of its roots, stem, foliage, and the bud itself at the level of their hearts. Their breath, their hugs and kisses, and their love encourage the lotus flower to blossom, and in this flower, their child is conceived. The presence of your future or already-born children can make this very simple part of the practice even more colorful, as the joyful laughter of children and their ability to fantasize and imagine is much brighter than it is in we adults.

---

*The five Ms refer to transgressive substances used in tantric rituals. They include *madya*, or wine-amrita; *mamsa*, or meat; *matsya*, which refers to two key prana energy channels in the body, the Ida and the Pingala, which are controlled by pranayama and are visualized as two structures of a figure-eight shape interwoven like two fish; *mudra* refers to sacred hand gestures that activate the kundalini energy; and *maithuna*, referring to sexual intercourse and female sexual discharge.

THE PHYSIOLOGY OF SEX

Let's dive a little deeper into the temple of our sexual nature, our physiological structure. These discoveries are the result of many years of scientific research as well as the experience of various tantric schools.

Nowadays, especially among middle-aged women, the demand to display overt sexuality has increased, which has led to a surge in certain professions such as sexual massage therapists, male strippers, men who perform cunnilingus and can get women to squirt, and even fellatio trainers. All this is understandable—the market responds to demand. These pleasures, if they are not a part of training for couples, are quite expensive. Delving into the cause of the inability to orgasm is very often quite a tedious process as some women are desperate to experience the pleasure about which so much is said.

But it turns out that the road to squirting does not lie in the hands of a trainer, but in the woman herself, in her trust in her own body and her ability to free her consciousness from constant control. A big part of orgasm is letting go of feelings of guilt and shame, usually acquired in childhood. A healthy body, even on a subconscious level, will tend to orgasm, and there is nothing shameful in this from the point of view of our physiology. However, when we were children, most likely the development of our libido was thwarted by social programming. Here is an example: A boy is caught masturbating by his grandmother, and not only does she shame him for it, she also punishes him by forbidding him to have any interaction with his friends. Then his mother, having learned about the incident from her mother, cancels their upcoming Sunday trip to the zoo. His father, though, laughs at the women and takes his son to the movies and buys him an ice cream and lemonade. As a result, the boy develops trust, including trust of his sexual nature, but only with men.

This example points to the root cause of female frigidity—shame and guilt. In many cases it also results in a person rejecting sexual attraction to the opposite sex. To feel pleasure, you need to create a space for it, both in your body and in your mind. If a woman hears about the

74 The Alchemy of Conception

vaunted multi-orgasm, she might get to thinking *What if it doesn't happen?* or *What if I can't?* These fears do not contribute to relaxation and to giving oneself over completely to both the process and the partner.

Marina's Field Notes

I had a case once where a woman had two children but had never climaxed. Sometimes, to avoid disappointing her husband, she would fake an orgasm, all the while assuring herself that just like her mother, she was simply incapable of achieving one. She became pregnant with her third child, and in an effort to give birth differently this time, she agreed to an erotic massage, for once forgetting her mother's moralistic legacy. Her husband wanted his wife to be healthy and wanted a happy baby, yet they had almost entirely stopped having sex after the first two children.

Of course, some preparatory work was in order, such as teaching them that sex is not forbidden during pregnancy, and that mastery in sex is something one must train in. I informed them about hormonal surges and the wonderful opportunity to find sexual harmony after childbirth. The husband diligently studied Taoist Healing Love practices and massages and started to do yoga and Chi Kung with his wife and two children. For the first time, the sex gates finally opened with delightful intercourse preceded by gentle erotic massage.

The resulting childbirth was a great proclamation of love creativity. Their third boy was born in orgasmic waters and received in the arms of his father. Their family happiness continues to this day. This couple now has seven children: six boys and one girl. The woman became a psychotherapist specializing in pregnancy and family relations, and the father, in addition to his main work, took up the art of photography. He lovingly filmed the birth and training of all their subsequent children. This further inspired him to make films about the early development of children.

This couple opened the door for me, too, inspiring me to realize that orgasmic childbirth isn't only for a select few, but for any pair of lovers who are trusting and determined to find this natural path of creative sexuality.

WOMAN, MAN, AND ORGASM

To better experience the alchemy of sexuality, it is important to study the structure of the organs in full detail and understand their mission in orgasm. An orgasm is an excitement that first begins in the head, producing appropriate hormones, exciting the blood and moving it from the erogenous zones to the sex organs, and from there, back to the glands and other organs. All this results in the ecstasy that brings on orgasm. In both the female and the male body, orgasm pours forth like a liquid in powerful vibrations of pleasure. This pleasure can be spilled and wasted, or it can be strengthened and prolonged.

Male orgasm consists of three parts: erection, friction, and ejaculation, and of course a prelude to arousal is required. Female orgasm is more complex and more spectacular. After gradual arousal, she reaches a plateau phase, and then she experiences possibly multiple innervations with orgasm, or reaches just the brink of orgasm. This is the resolution of the plateau phase—the ability to relax when

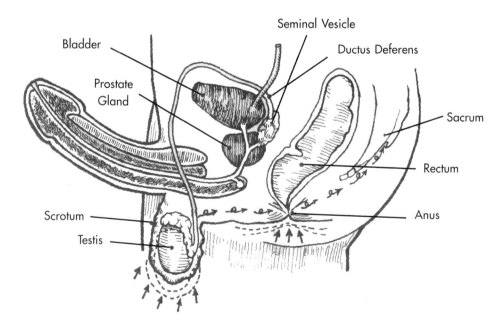

Fig. 3.5. Male reproductive organs

strongly aroused—that can feel like a prolonged orgasm that slowly spreads throughout the entire body. Can these two processes happen simultaneously?

It would seem that for men everything is simple and in plain sight. But it is no coincidence that the prostate gland is located deep inside a man and is attached to his bladder. The urethra passes through the prostate, the center of male pleasure being the vas deferens, sometimes called the sperm duct. The number of prostate spasms and the quality and duration of pleasure depends on the man's muscle strength and blood supply. The head of the penis is connected to its body, and the root goes down, delving into his crotch, continuing down to the middle of the scrotum, dividing it into two parts, where the balls "float." Then the muscle of the perineum connects with the external and internal sphincter of the anus. All these areas contain many erogenous zones. The Jade Wand—the penis—is itself very emotional. It creates a rush of blood that fills the organ all the way to the tip of the wand, where the opening there produces secretions to ensure good passage for sperm. The ejaculatory ducts that flow into the male urethra are quite long, each duct being about 40 cm, while the total length of the sperm "road" from the right and left testicles through the bladder and prostate gland is 80 cm. The sperm must make their way along this route, filling up with an elixir of prostate secretions and lubrication as they do. Part of the lubrication is produced before ejaculation. These secretions dilute the denser semen, creating conditions for the sperm to get through the urinary tract and up into the female vagina, protecting the semen in its new habitat. The enriched sperm, when it connects with the female ejaculation, or amrita, turns into the Elixir of Immortality, useful both for conception and for high pleasure.

The female vagina is designed for pleasure, and for the birth of a child. When a man enters her secret gate, the engorged ring of her outer vaginal muscles clench around his blood-filled penis, and as liquid is pushed out of the crown of his penis, it mixes with her vaginal waters. As the penis slides in and rubs against the walls of the vagina, her cervix swells, followed by culmination or prolongation.

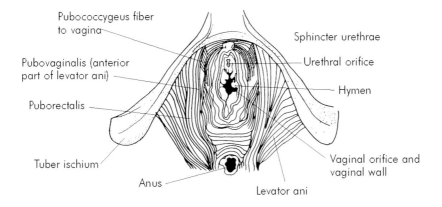

Fig. 3.6. The "love muscle" includes the pubococcygeus (PC muscle), pubovaginalis, and puborectalis.

The man is overcome by orgasmic contractions due to the release of lubricant and friction of the phallus in the vagina. The peak comes for him when the prostate enters the phase of spontaneous contractions—the point of no return—and sperm passes through the prostate, to which the vagina usually reacts with suction vibrations. Good and long orgasm is achieved not only as a result of excellent health, but through the synchronization of the partners. A man should not immediately enter deeply; he should push his climactic erection at the upper vault of the vagina, which can create multi-orgasmic sensations of female squirting. The secret is the fast and slow pushes when sliding in and out—this way the male phallus arouses all the erogenous zones connected to the woman's urethral sponge in the upper vault. Orgasms are triggered by the very thin and sensitive venous plexus of the woman's Skene's glands—the quality of orgasm depending on the amount of fluid.

Let's now consider the woman's secret cave. What does this flower, which resembles an orchid, consist of? Pulling the outer lips apart, we see the hooded head of the clitoris that continues down to the butterfly-shaped inner lips. The head of the clitoris is a part of the body of the clitoris, and on both sides are the bulbs of the opening and the Bartholin's glands that pass their ducts through the outer lips and connect to the inner structure. The body of the clitoris divides into two "legs" that go deep into the labia; the ducts of the glands are deep inside this tissue and are extremely thin—they intertwine with the veins and go around the urethra. The female urethra is only 3 cm long, which makes it very vulnerable and not always capable of holding in pee, especially during pregnancy and after childbirth.

Next we see the opening of the vagina, followed by the perineum and the anus. Going deeper into the "cave," we can now examine its vaults. Here is the area of the urethral sponge and the G-spot, located on the pistil of the upper vault. The lower vault is joined with the perineum by the muscles and is very close to the rectum and its sphincters. The vaginal canal has muscle rings that can flex and relax. The upper ring is connected to the opening of the cervix and its hood, which also swells with stimulation. Then there's the cervix itself, which turns into the uterus and two ovaries with ducts that lead to the layered epithelium of the uterus. Inside the ovaries are the woman's eggs, each egg a hundred times larger than a single sperm.

And so the couple's eyes meet, their breathing hastens, their lips meet, their bodies entwine in an embrace. Usually, the woman will feel swelling in her breasts and in the perineum area, and a tickling sensation starts in her coccyx and in her legs, or electricity runs down to her abdomen. The man will have two streams of blood set off by veins and arteries, filling the cavernous and spongy bodies of his sexual organs. Gentle touches and kisses make the swollen head of the penis go up under the pressure of desire and blood. The foreskin stretches over the body of the penis, the scrotum tenses and rises, and the phallus is ready to penetrate.

For the woman, this phase of desire becomes arousal. Her excitation is especially heightened when her nipples and labia are touched. Blood flow and spasms affect the area of the female "prostate," the rudimentary organ that is stored behind the Skene's glands, located around the lower end of the urethra. This female prostate is formed while she is a fetus, and eventually remains, but as a rudimentary organ, never developing into a full male prostate. Nevertheless, this area retains a sensitive connection with the Skene's glands and nerves and is very reactive to arousal, promoting the release of lubrication. Swelling up, the outer labia parts like flower petals under the weight of raindrops to reveal the glistening clitoris head. The bulbs of the clitoral threshold are also engorged as well as the "legs" of the clitoris as they press on the venous plexus and the Bartholin's gland to create a semblance of ejaculation, emitting two milliliters of viscous lubricant white in color that covers the entrance to the vagina and remains unabsorbed for quite some time. Strong swelling makes the vagina elastic. The tissues of the perineum and the body of the clitoris press on the urethra and the first third of the vagina, along with the urethral sponge.

At this time, the male crown, with the so-called bulbous glands, similar to the Bartholin's glands, begin to secrete lubricant. The human body is very concerned with healthy reproduction, so it provides sperm as well as a vitamin cocktail of prostate secretions, seminal vesicles, and bulbous duct lubrication. Male orgasm as well as female is subject to remission. When the phallus enters the secret gate, the vagina spasms at this entrance with the rush of blood. The hood of the clitoris pulls back, the head of the clitoris becomes erect, and the glands create additional lubrication. Contractions of the uterus turn the cervix from the anus to the vagina. The vagina lengthens, the cervix straightens, and the uterus is pulled up. Inside the vagina, sperm acquires a proper consistency to penetrate the fallopian tubes and zealously moves on to meet a possible egg. At the same time, when the woman is in the plateau phase and if she does not fall into the resolution, she will continue on her way to conception.

What stands in the way of female orgasm? Possibly, a strong negative attachment to it. The memory of childish masturbation can also be one of the reasons why women struggle to orgasm with a man. A child's orgasm is an unconscious pleasure that a girl usually receives when defecating or urinating.* Unconscious sexuality is activated at

---

*A diaper contributes to the dullness of the sensations in the genital area of a baby and to muscle weakness, as there is no need to complete the process with multiple attempts and pushes that train the genital muscles.

about three years of age, and girls who are capable of fantasy and associative thinking quickly learn to experience a sharp and pleasant sensation when touching their genitals. When masturbation occurs easily and simply (even without bodily contact), which is recorded by the limbic system, the brain evaluates the information and does not allow it to go any further to a more complex process if the girl's sexual imprinting has been colored by the moralistic judgments of society around sexuality.

Great expectations of love with a man in a sexual partnership are crushed against this kind of childhood matrix. The girl whose sexuality has been thwarted does not think that it is worth considering her own needs and getting a new, more satisfying sexual experience, one that allows her to orgasm.

FEMALE EJACULATION AND THE G-SPOT

Gynecology as a science states that there are no erectile organs in a woman and not so many nerve plexuses in the upper vault of the birth canal, which makes the birth of a child easier (less blood and pain). We disagree, and so do many sexologists. Studies on the female erectile organs and glands have finally cracked the mystery of the G-spot. This is confirmed by our observations of natural childbirth outside the hospital (freebirth) and especially in water childbirth. The phallus or fingers (or even the more voluminous head of the baby making pressing movements as it pulls to the exit), together with the vibrations of the woman as the erogenous zones of her vagina are engorged with blood, bring her to arousal. Her energy is at the peak of resolution at this point, and she ejaculates as the Skene's glands of the urethral sponge gush out sweet, transparent liquid rich in microelements. This liquid is the primary urine produced by the kidneys, intended to be absorbed by the blood. It is a concentrated product emitted from all the bodily fluids into the blood (120–70 liters passing through the kidneys daily), containing many substances, including hormones that can be lost along with blood waste. The arousal and resolution of this phase of female ejaculation is called *brain orgasm, hypothalamic orgasm, neotomic orgasm, dark orgasm,* or *wet orgasm.* More commonly we know it as squirting.

To achieve squirting that is not spontaneous as it is in natural childbirth, the woman must accept its existence and be able to relax at the very beginning of erotic massage, even though there may be some possibly not entirely comfortable sensations. You need trust, good-quality oil, and not being afraid to let go or push out when the need to urinate comes. This is the second female ejaculation with an interesting, muted orgasm prolonged to infinity that comes with the *feeling* of needing to go to the toilet, then comes relaxation, tension, relaxation again, and eventually climax. The question arises as to whether an unspontaneous, provoked squirting is good for you?

There is no definitive answer. We let out the liquid that should become a component of our blood with its many necessary elements. Of course it can be replenished. The woman should drink plenty of water, as we all should, to ensure proper hydration, a necessity in female ejaculation. If you would like to try this extraordinary pleasure, you will need to train the muscles of the vagina and the diaphragm. The Yoni Egg practice (see chapter 1) is good training for this, as well as training to hold in and then release a strong flow when urinating. Kegel exercises are also a good way to naturally train the vaginal muscles. Otherwise, the orgasmic capability will weaken (just as it will in men who frequently ejaculate) and muscle lethargy will start to take place. Women have a very short and not very strong urethra with its sphincters, which is why sometimes a woman cannot hold her urine in. Squirting is directly related to this duct and the muscles around it, so don't overwork them. In addition, sex offers a strong hormonal surge, and in this case an excessive release of vasopressin is required to restore the function of the hypothalamus, which is always involved in our libido. Squirting can be called a hypothalamic deviation from the process of dividing the blood in the kidneys and throwing out its useful part, instead of absorbing it back into the blood. This gets the hypothalamus confused. For its rapid recovery, vasopressin, which is similar in properties to oxytocin, is appropriate here, and both are associated with love.

82   The Alchemy of Conception

If you overdo sex, this kind of hypersexuality can disrupt the function of the hypothalamus. So if you decide to use this way of relieving stress, then you should treat squirting as a festive ritual to relieve any tension in your relationship. Interestingly, immediately after this exotic pleasure, the sexual appetite increases, so squirting can be a prelude to intercourse.

We teach this exotic technique to couples and sometimes use the same kind of erotic massage to relax before childbirth, or after. (It is better when this is taught to both partners, but sadly not all future dads are open to intimacy during pregnancy and immediately afterward.) Creativity is always necessary in a loving relationship. Squirting can exacerbate diseases of the genitourinary system due to the increase of the blood flow, but it cannot cause permanent harm. Should any symptoms arise, they are simply revealing an already existing condition, and this gives the woman a chance to work on it. If there is fungus in the vagina, for example, the sensations provided by the fingers can be both pleasant and painful. Therefore it is advised to wash the birth canal when aroused. It is better to use natural solutions with the necessary flora—yogurt diluted with water works really well. If you have any doubts, consult a competent doctor and follow their directions before starting to squirt.

Many men do not realize that their health and creativity show up not only in the regulation of their own ejaculation, but also in that of the woman, in her truly mystical waters, so rich in minerals. To get to these gems and cut them into diamonds of health, you need to become a master who knows and accepts his wealth. A man should take care of the health of his prostate and check for inflammation, either with the help of a good doctor or by learning from a master how to examine himself during self-massage.

The G-spot is also connected to certain sensations in the perineum and anus, since the nerve and venous plexuses pass from the erogenous zones of the vagina through the perineum to the anus. When we stretch the lower vault (the inner muscle of the female perineum) with the fingers, we come into contact with the mystical and secret area of the Hui

Yin (located at the very root of the torso, at the center of the pelvic floor, a half inch in front of the anus). Some women experience very strong orgasmic vibrations when this area is stimulated through the anus. The erogenous nerves of the clitoris connect with the anal sphincter. In erotic massage, this area is engaged through the massage of the buttocks (which contain four very sensual points), especially the area at their base. But not everyone is open to these intimate interactions, and most people don't even suspect the larger possibilities of orgasm. Once again, we would like to remind you that a prolonged orgasm consisting of strong spasmodic vibrations is a sensation experienced by all the sex organs and their glands, ducts, and bulbs. It is quite possible that modern sexologists are right when they say that there are no orgasms of different areas: the clitoris, vagina, and uterus create a single intelligent orgasm that rises to the heart through all the nerve plexuses and organs, leaving the vibrations of love in the body for a long time, until the next intercourse. Sensual love is like the sounds of a gong that has just been rung. It creates extraordinarily beautiful and long-lasting sounds, delighting the ears and harmonizing the surrounding space.

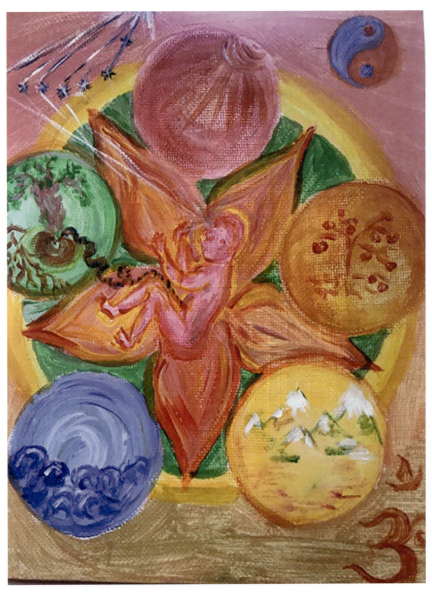

Illustration by Marina Dadasheva-Drown

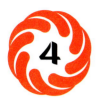

4

Pregnancy

The first and main source of our happiness is our mother. The zygote becomes an embryo that emerges because of sexual interaction and becomes the fruit of love. In humans, the embryo is identical in its initial form to the developing embryos of many other mammals. Gradually, though, the human-to-be acquires very significant differences as the transformation from two cells meeting and greeting to a conscious living human being progresses, until we finally get to meet the magical child.

At first, the in-utero child senses the world through the mother's perception of life. By the fifth month, the baby has acquired seven senses: touch, hearing, sight, taste, and smell, plus the vestibular sense, which governs balance and movement, and proprioception, the sense of knowing where a body part is without looking at it, as well as five more subtle chakras. By the seventh month the baby can recognize its mother's moods and has acquired the ability to evaluate via the neocortex. The unborn child begins to feel the vibrations of sounds and colors as well. Psychiatrist Thomas Verny, who has studied and written extensively about the "embodied mind" (the title of one of his books), says:

> The great weight of the scientific evidence that has emerged over the last decade demands that we reevaluate the mental and emotional abilities of unborn children. Awake or asleep, the studies show, they

86 Pregnancy

[unborn children] are constantly tuned in to their mother's every action, thought, and feeling. From the moment of conception, the experience in the womb shapes the brain and lays the groundwork for personality, emotional temperament, and the power of higher thought.[1]

Anything that does not correspond to the natural impulses of life inside the mother is difficult to process for the not yet fully formed brain of the tiny human, who relies on the intuitive impulses of its heart, whose sacred cells hold a memory identical to the memory of the ancient brain. An esoteric understanding of our biological structure suggests that these cells in the heart are where the individual human soul settles.

We can only guess at how the developing fetus feels upon being subjected to an ultrasound, which probably feels like an invasion, as most ultrasound transducers in current use operate at very high frequency, in the megahertz (MH_z) range. Ultrasound invasion does not correspond with the much lower natural vibrations of the human body and violates the intimacy of the baby. One shouldn't challenge the logic behind the natural development of the spiritual and emotional qualities of a person just to satisfy one's curiosity about the gender of the baby.

CONNECTING WITH THE INNER SMILE AND SIX HEALING SOUNDS

The Inner Smile meditation (see chapter 2) engaged in relation to both you and the baby's organs found in chapter 2, along with the Six Healing Sounds, described below, are wonderful ways to establish the positive qualities of the organs both in yourself and in your baby.

The Inner Smile practice, when sent to the baby, unites mother and child in a smile to each of the organs; this cultivates the virtues of these organs, along with absolute health. This is a wonderful way to build a loving foundation of health and vitality for your gestating human. The mother smiles to her heart, filling it with all the necessary elements

Pregnancy   87

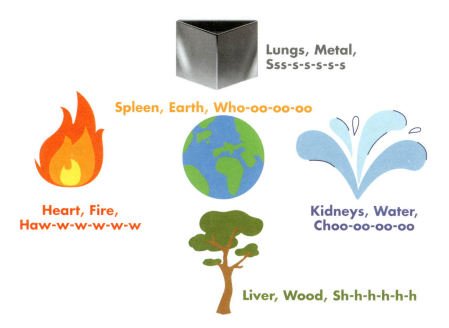

Fig. 4.1. Five of the six healing sounds. The Triple Warmer is not shown because it is a balancing and finishing sound and as such is not associated with any element or color. The Triple Warmer's sound is hee-e-e-e-e.

and qualities; she then smiles at the heart of her baby with her heart, connecting with the delicate feeling of love in the child's heart. After the birth of the child this will help the mother intuitively understand, for example, the reason why the baby cries, whether due to hunger, a tummy ache, needing a diaper change, or wanting to sleep. This heart connection will also set the foundation for their future lives together. The Inner Smile meditation is also offered to those who just before conception want to create the prototype for a healthy baby. In other words, we call in the soul of the child and build a temple for it.

The Six Healing Sounds meditation* is a beautiful ritual that includes slow, mindful breathing, visualization of the organs, and, of course, the six sounds that correspond to the organs. This meditation

---

*For a more detailed description of this practice, see also Master Chia's book *Chi Kung for Radiant Skin* (Destiny Books, 2022), pp. 128–39.

creates a wonderful state of relaxation and calm for both mother and child, especially when done before going to bed, as it will lead to a beautiful, deep, restful sleep. Once the steps are memorized it is not always necessary to go through every organ; you can practice on individual organs, such as the heart, which is especially beneficial for connecting with the love energy of your baby. All the sounds are barely audible and produced on a long, slow exhalation at the level of a whisper.

All of these sounds can be done while seated; the Triple Warmer sound at the conclusion can be done either seated or lying down.

The Six Healing Sounds

Lungs
Sss-s-s-s-s-s

Healing sounds sent to the lungs instill the positive energies of courage, justice, and righteousness in you and your baby.

1. Sit straight on the edge of a chair. Plant both feet on the floor. Imagine your feet are growing roots and connecting you to the earth.
2. Take a deep breath and slowly let it out. Relax.
3. Gently rock your spine side to side, starting from the base of your spine and gradually progressing to the neck area. As you rock your spine, imagine a fiery dragon swimming up your spine, enlivening and energizing it.
4. Feel your baby as a source of loving energy. When you start feeling that love, smile. Imagine your smile as being sunshine warming the surface of a lake. Feel that sunshine entering your baby's heart and reflecting that love back to you.
5. Bring your attention to your lungs. Smile into your lungs. See your lungs filling with white light. Place your hands near your lungs, palms facing the lungs. Feel their energy. Smile and send this energy to your baby's lungs.

6. To produce the lung's sound, inhale, smile slightly, put your tongue behind your teeth and let the hissing sound, sss-s-s-s-s, emerge on a long, slow exhale with little effort. It is not a loud sound, but rather a quiet, snakelike hiss. Smile and send this sound to your baby's lungs.

Kidneys
Choo-oo-oo-oo

Healing sounds sent to the kidneys dissipate any fears lodged there and instill in you and your baby the positive virtues of stillness, tranquility, and gentleness.

1. Bring your attention to your kidneys. Become aware of the watery energy of the kidneys. Smile into your kidneys. Fill your kidneys with deep blue light.
2. As you smile into your kidneys, smile into the kidneys of your baby, filling them with the same deep blue light and the element of water.
3. Rub your hands together to warm them and place your hands on the kidney area on your back. Inhale, round your lips, and then as you exhale, produce the kidney's sound softly: choo-oo-oo-oo. Send the sound to your baby's kidneys, along with the virtues of that organ—calmness, tranquility, and gentleness.

Liver
Sh-h-h-h-h-h

The liver's sound clears negative energies in you such as anger or guilt and instills in you and your baby the positive energies of kindness, forgiveness, and generosity.

1. Bring your attention to your liver. Smile into your liver. Become aware of the energy of the liver, and fill it with the warm, earthy green of the wood element.

90   Pregnancy

2. As you smile into your liver, smile into the liver of your baby, filling your baby's liver with the same warm, earthy green color.

3. Rub your hands together to warm them and place them over your liver. Inhale and slowly exhale, producing the liver's sound, sh-h-h-h-h-h, as if you wanted to hush someone. Send the sound to your baby's liver, along with the virtues of that organ—kindness, forgiveness, and generosity.

♺ Heart
Haw-w-w-w-w-w

The heart's sound instills the positive energies of love, joy, patience, and happiness in you and your baby.

1. Bring your attention to your heart. Place your palms over your heart. Feel the energy of the heart. Smile into your heart. Become aware of the energy of the heart and fill it with the warm, red energy of the element of fire.

2. As you smile into your heart, smile into the heart of your baby, filling your baby's heart with the same warm energy of the element of fire.

3. Inhale, then open and round your lips, forming the sound of *h* as in *heart*, then continue with a long exhalation as if expressing a sigh of relief, haw-w-w-w-w-w. Send the heart's sound, haw-w-w-w-w-w, to your baby's heart, along with the virtues of that organ—love, joy, patience, and happiness.

♺ Spleen
Who-oo-oo-oo

The spleen's sound dissipates worry and instills the positive energies of trust, confidence, fairness, openness, and faith in you and your baby.

1. Bring your attention to your spleen. Become aware of the energy of your spleen. Hold your palms facing your spleen. Smile into your spleen. Fill your spleen with the yellow light of the element of earth.

Pregnancy **91**

2. As you smile into your spleen, smile into your baby's spleen, filling it with the same yellow energy of the element of earth.
3. Inhale, form the sound of the letter *w*, and proceed with the spleen's sound, who-oo-oo-oo, like an owl, produced on a long, slow exhalation. Smile and send the spleen's sound to your baby's spleen, along with the virtues of that organ—trust, confidence, fairness, openness, and faith.

Triple Warmer
Hee-e-e-e-e

The Triple Warmer is an acupuncture meridian that involves the thyroid, thymus, and adrenal glands and controls the fight-flight-freeze response. Its sound balances the temperature of the upper warmer (the area above the diaphragm, which often gets very hot due to intense metabolic activity), the middle warmer (the area between the diaphragm and the navel, where the digestive organs are located and which often has slower metabolism, especially if a person is leading a sedentary lifestyle), and the lower warmer (location of the reproductive organs and organs responsible for elimination of waste, which often get too cold and need warming up). The Triple Warmer's sound helps to distribute heat evenly throughout the body. This sound is different from the other organ sounds because it is not connected to any particular emotion, color, or element. It is a finishing sound that balances all six sounds in both you and your baby, so it's a great finale to this practice.

1. For this sound, get into a lying-down position or continue to sit comfortably in a chair.
2. Raise your arms overhead and smile. Include your baby in that smile, imaging your baby's Triple Warmer meridian receiving that smile.
3. Repeat this gesture three times. Visualize any excess heat leaving your body and your baby's body.
4. Inhale, form the sound of the letter *h*, then release the Triple Warmer's sound, hee-e-e-e-e-e, on a long, slow exhalation, as in *leap* or *heap*. Smile and send this sound to you and your baby.

PREPARING FOR BREAST-FEEDING

We strongly advise women who lost their breast milk before nursing commences or whose baby refused to breast-feed in the beginning to give extra special attention to bonding. Ask yourself what emotions contradict love and replace them with positive ones. It may be the fear of losing your milk or your husband's attention, a fear that you'll ruin the shape of your breasts with breast-feeding, or anxiety about the family's future related to your financial situation. The Inner Smile and the Six Healing Sounds will help the organs that are directly responsible for each emotion. Fear is associated with the kidneys and the genitourinary system, so make the sound of this organ as often as possible: choo-oo-oo-oo, similar to the sound a train or the wind makes. Think about the calm blueness of the ocean or a quiet pond. Imagine the reflection of the bright sun in the water and be filled with softness and tenderness, and then convey this feeling to your baby and its father.

Prepare for the breast-feeding journey with pleasure by doing the breast massage outlined in chapter 1, "Warming the Breasts." Massage thirty-six times toward the inside and thirty-six times toward the outside around both of your breasts using both of your hands. You can add an element of erotica to it by inviting your partner to participate in this massage. The mystical animal that supports the state of happiness in the genitourinary system is the Black Tortoise, and the protector of the kidneys is the Blue Deer.

Visualizing and trusting the images of these mystical animals will calm the mind. Anxiety is common among all expectant parents. According to the Universal Healing Tao, the spleen (not only the heart) is responsible for jump-starting the period of being parents. This is where all the anxiety is stored. Concentrate on trust and openness. These are the virtues of the spleen, the stomach, and the pancreas. With a smile, let bright golden sunrays into these organs; let these rays reflect in the water along with the image of a sunflower. Remember the taste of sweet apples in the fall and call to your side the Yellow Phoenix to be your guardian and supporter. For a parent it is extremely useful

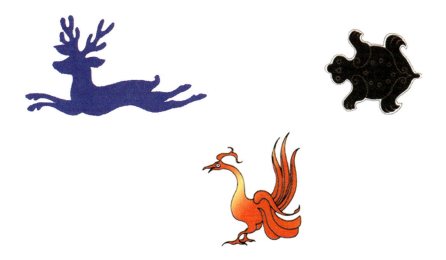

Fig. 4.2. Blue Deer, Yellow Phoenix, Black Turtle

to develop your imagination in a way that accords with the fabulous images of childhood. More visualizations and trust! And let us not forget about the sexual aspect of lactation. By increasing your libido, you increase the release of all the hormones associated with love and pleasure, including oxytocin and prolactin, which get transferred to your nursing baby.

Any misconception that the sexual properties of hormones are suppressed by breast-feeding most likely stems from the first days after birth, when a woman with tender and unprepared breasts finds it painful to feed her baby. In a healthy newborn, the sucking reflex is very strong, so the breasts must be prepared for this onslaught. Nipple massage without oil, pulling at them, pinching them, and so forth helps the skin toughen and prevents injury. Bras need to be roomy and made of natural material, flax or cotton, and not press on the mammary glands. In addition to breast massage, we recommend pouring cold water over your body starting with your head, getting out in the fresh air from the first day after birth, and letting the indoors be filled with as much light as possible as well as fresh air, for air baths for the breasts. Sleeping in a bra or wearing any kind of clothing to bed is not recommended;

94   Pregnancy

the stagnation of milk as well as continuous pumping can easily lead to infectious mastitis. Aside from regular breast care, be sure to change positions when feeding to allow the outflow of milk from all parts of the mammary glands. This helps ensure the health of the baby and the mother, which also benefits the marriage.

INSTILLING LOVE AND TRUST

The spirit is found through the womb; the soul comes into it. This theme has been developed in the books of Joseph Chilton Pearce (1926–2016), who has written extensively on human development. Pearce stresses the importance of preserving transcendental abilities in a person, starting with conception and continuing through all stages of development. The biggest problem, according to Pearce, is that a child's loss of his individuality and transcendent capabilities stems from society's system of prohibitions and taboos. Guilt and shame replace the natural human urge to be aware and awake and contribute to the dissolution of the anterior lobes of a child's brain, which thereafter absorb society's inhibitions and suppressions. A human being needs to live out his or her potential at all levels of existence. Our physiological body is a vessel for energies by which we acquire spirituality and knowledge. Different parts of the brain are responsible for different functions of human existence. Restrictions in communication with parents or peers, other species, or the opposite sex, and prohibitions against certain forms of touch and taste as well as these kinds of interactions with animals and plants minimize the functioning of a child's brain and narrow the child's attention span as well as the scope of possible actions. These restrictions are artificially created by the medical system as early as during the fetal development stage. This system views pregnancy as a disease and therefore a pregnant woman should not be allowed the natural joys of life, like riding a bike, doing sports, actively moving, and eating whatever the body is asking for. The most ridiculous restriction of all is the one that recommends that pregnant women not make love—the very origin of her pregnancy! Through that last restriction, the child while still in the womb loses touch with his father and often feels as though he's divided between his parents later in life.

Many people have consciously returned to these primal memories in sessions of rebirthing and holotropic breath work, which are described in the books of Stanislav Grof, one of the principal developers of transpersonal psychology. Grof maintains that "the assignment of an individual spiritual entity to a particular physical body occurs during conception according to its karmic past; this choice bypasses the laws of heredity and genetics."[2] In moments of altered consciousness produced through rhythmic cyclic breathing, a person can return to her subconscious and explore it and even alter it so as not to repeat past negative situations, and importantly, not pass them on to her children. Sometimes you can trace the behavioral patterns of a mother in her daughter's future sex life to account for such things as alienation from the father and growing up in a single-parent family. Since usually a woman gives birth to her first child the same way her mother gave birth to her, if you enter the subconscious before or during pregnancy and replace this negative experience with a positive one, it will not have to be repeated in the present. For example, a woman can change the traumatic experience of the mother who gave birth to her through a cesarean section. For both the woman and her future child, this represents a release from the unnatural matrix and opens a door to innumerable creative possibilities.

Nowadays there isn't enough common knowledge about the origin of a human being and the cellular memory of the heart, as well as the spectacular release of love hormones during pregnancy, so these hormones get unconsciously suppressed during pregnancy and childbirth. As a result, the child grows up in a deficit of love. Childbirth today is not considered to be the apotheosis of a sexual and loving relationship, but rather a surgical procedure with epidural intervention, which deenergizes and immobilizes the woman's womb. And if a woman does manage to avoid a C-section, this is what the medical system calls "natural" childbirth.

What about the child's first knowledge of sex, which occurs at the time of birth? We already know what awaits these children in the future. People who were born in an unnatural way end up being limited in their emotional resources due to the traumatic experience of their birth, during which time the emotions and attitudes that were planted during conception and immediately afterward got established. Taoists believe that compassion is a mixture of all human virtues. It consists of everything related to love: kindness, sensitivity, courage, respect, justice—all of them blended into one, like a compote made from different berries. Since virtues exist in different proportions within each person, people experience happiness in different ways. Compassion cannot be obtained from just one ingredient. Same as compote—it cannot become sweet if you only use sour berries; you must add sugar or other ingredients to sweeten it.

Positive qualities are created by the five elements: fire, water, metal, wood, and earth. These elements comprise a cycle of mutual help in their constant transformation, in which each element becomes the progenitor of another. As a result, the creative circle of virtues is never exhausted, as it is created by the balance of yin and yang interactions. Thanks to water, the earth sprouts grain; the fire energy of the sun helps it grow out of the earth, blossom, and produce new seeds; the old tree burns down by the fire, and the ashes become a fertilizer for the soil; the earth forms minerals (the element of metal) that help in the cycle of transformation. To create and transform virtues, one must respect and understand the laws of nature and the relationship between the five elements.

Through loving compassion, the seed of life is laid, and it must go through its natural cycle: conception, pregnancy, birth, feeding, and training in the virtuous cycle. A mother who chooses epidural therapy or a cesarean section is robbing her child of a certain part of the journey. In his book *Pedagogia ontopsicologica* (Ontopsychological Pedagogy), Italian philosopher and artist Antonio Meneghetti, who founded the Ontopsychological school of psychology,* brings up the fact that during the nine months of pregnancy, a child is both part of the mother's body and its own independent self.

---

*A branch of psychology that sees the final goal of psychological knowledge as perfecting the human being and human society.

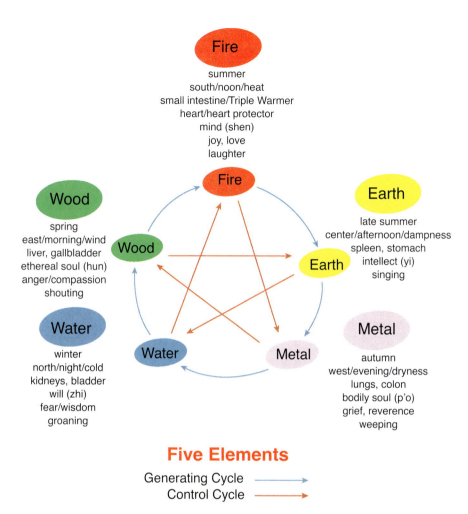

Fig. 4.3. The five major organs and their connection to the five elements

The child is part of the mother because it is part of her body, yet from the moment of fertilization we are already talking about an In-se. Meneghetti believes that throughout her pregnancy, a woman must perceive her child as a complete person, without falling into egoism, self-pity, or resentment, because these kinds of states can cause negative consequences of a psychotropic nature in the ethereal field of the child.

Stanislav Grof, in *Realms of the Human Unconscious*, considers this to be proof of the presence of both an individual and a collective

98   Pregnancy

memory inherent in the structure of the human subconscious. Motherhood requires deep awareness, not just the nurturing of the fetus. The Tao says that from the very moment of the origin of the zygote, the experiences of the mother affect the physical, spiritual, and emotional qualities of the developing fetus. This is why we offer expectant mothers and fathers wonderful meditations of the Universal Healing Tao.*

Carlos Castaneda's teacher, Don Juan, tells him that inside each person's individual cocoon of light there is a special place, the assemblage point, which governs one's ability to see the visible and the invisible and to hear what is audible and inaudible. In short, the location of this point determines one's reality. Given that in adults this point is already fixed due to deeply rooted impressions, an adult sees the world in a much narrower range in contrast to a child. As the child's assemblage point isn't yet fixed, it freely moves in the everyday world as well as the divine continuum. That's why a child can see the world more imaginatively and with a different range of sensations. Gradually the assemblage point stops moving and the child simply becomes an adult who has lost the original vision of the magical world, which Castaneda calls the "true" way of seeing. The ability to see and listen with the transcendent brain gradually dissolves as a child learns purely physical skills so as to adapt to life. During this extremely important time, the child's socialization takes place. Her world now encompasses a forbidden zone consisting of "no" and "not allowed." During this early stage of development, the child sees the world through her mother as she seeks her approval and support in her exploration of the environment; in so doing she is given constant prohibitions and restrictions that shut her world off to further observation and curiosity.

---

*A very creative and practical series of Taoist meditations are the Fusion Formulas, in which we neutralize our stimuli (irritants), taking them out of our organs and moving them to a number of small areas located nearby. In these "points" we mix negative qualities with virtues. After mixing, we cultivate the virtues and put them back into the organs. From the increased virtues we create a light pearl, and then use it to purify the channels of our physical and spiritual bodies. This is the subject of an entire book by Master Chia, *Fusion of the Five Elements* (Destiny Books, 1985, 2007).

Our parental choice is twofold: we can choose to raise a convenient, obedient child, managed through rules and "you cant's," or we can become an "inconvenient" parent in the eyes of the society and give our child smiles and laughter and freedom to explore their very humanness. Joseph Chilton Pearce, in *The Biology of Transcendence*, confirms this with a quote from American neuropsychologist Allan Schore, who says that "interactions with the mother directly influence the growth and assembly of the brain's structural systems that perform self-regulatory functions in the child . . . and mediate the individual interpersonal and intra-personal processes for life."[3]

It is hard to imagine how human cells respond to thoughts and images. In Taoist practice related to pregnancy, there are many examples confirming that love and trust can change the biological body and can influence the unborn child's decision to leave or stay. Quite often we have found that women who unconditionally trust their motherhood experience this as a salvation.

Marina's Field Notes

This incident took place almost thirty years ago, when I assisted a mother who was struggling to carry her child to full term.

I was approached by a woman named Svetlana, who was in the last trimester of pregnancy. She was frantic and in despair as she could no longer feel the movement of her baby. On that same day I turned to her doctor, who categorically stated that the fetus had stopped developing. He wanted to induce labor and terminate the pregnancy. Svetlana was in a daze, screaming and crying. As her spiritual midwife, I took her hand, looked into her eyes, and said that her heart was beating in unison with her child's heart, as that is exactly what I intuited. "Connect with him, feel the pulsation!" I told her. What was happening? Maybe the baby was hiding before birth and didn't want any outside interference. "Talk to him, persuade him to come back, tell him! Imagine how good it will be for you two to be together." That was the first step. The second: I asked her to feel the baby's micro-breathing in the water

100   Pregnancy

through her own matrix. We went to a pool and began to dive together, breathing rhythmically: inhaling above the water, exhaling under. The goal was to enter deep into the subconscious sense of faith and trust, to feel the child's life as her own, and to match her biorhythm with the baby's. We dived like this for half an hour, and afterward she said with a smile that she felt kicking, and on the left side of her abdomen we saw a bulge. That was part of the victory! But we still had to secure it.

The woman happily agreed to my suggestion to go to her husband and let him feel the heartbeat of the baby. "Is it a boy?" she asked. I confirmed what my intuition and my practical experience had told me, but she nevertheless hesitated. "My husband didn't believe me and sent me to the doctor for an ultrasound. It's scheduled for tomorrow." She didn't want to do it but had agreed to do so to avoid conflict with her husband. In our childbirth group, ultrasound is not recommended, as it takes away from the baby's sense of trust, which is important to cultivate at this stage. We prefer to wait patiently for whoever is to come and not interfere in the sacred life of the baby with mechanical interventions like this. In her personal beliefs, Svetlana was against any interference in the intimacy of the pregnancy.

Her husband did not want to go to our group preparation for childbirth, and Svetlana did not want to attend the group alone. After communicating with the baby, both future parents realized that the child could abandon them at any time if they were not in solidarity and did not listen to the baby's choices. All children are different, and sometimes they come as teachers.

Later, the parents happily got acquainted with the energy and physiology of the formation and birth of a person. They learned to understand their firstborn by bonding with the spirit of the developing baby. They began to study the effects of acupuncture on the biorhythm of labor, and they mastered the art of intimate massage and stroking the tummy along with singing songs and telling fairy tales to the unborn child. The three of them started going to symphony concerts and exhibitions; they read spiritual books, and they learned yoga and gymnastics; Chi Kung practices entered their lives a few years later and became a great help.

I was there during the birth. Like many children, Ivan was born into the loving embrace and kisses of his parents. Smiling, he emerged from the waters of his mother following a water birth and immediately took to the breast. Five minutes later, his old home, the placenta, floated out, everything happening in harmony, without fear, only love! Three days later, when the umbilical cord fell away from the beautiful umbilical ring by itself, the family went to a sauna with an ice fountain, where the baby learned to be strong and healthy in courageous solidarity with his parents.

The duality of the child with the mother remains while it's needed, to about two to three years of age. This is the period of forming basic adaptive skills. The libido is activated during peristalsis as the child learns to flex its urogenital muscle; breast-feeding also has an effect on this activation.

In Hinduism, the concept of *moksha*, or ultimate liberation, is about gaining freedom from reincarnation. It's important for us to understand, however, that this is not our choice. When we return it does not happen because we want to, and the same is true when we stop returning. Chinese wisdom says that the body is a great gift to the soul, and the road of the body to finding the soul is not easy. The soul is called and given permission, then conception happens, then pregnancy and birth, and then comes breast-feeding, overcoming the difficulties of growing up, and after all of that, the personality is released into a world of challenging situations and difficult people. A person needs to acquire the necessary life experience for the creation of the life path and its purpose.

STAGES OF FETAL DEVELOPMENT

A still mind, without evaluations or judgments, is called meditation, and a pregnant woman has the ability to be constantly in this state. She needs to understand that her child is her main teacher and guide during pregnancy. We also must remember that starting at twelve weeks, all the systems in the baby's body are functional—it is a human with a

102 Pregnancy

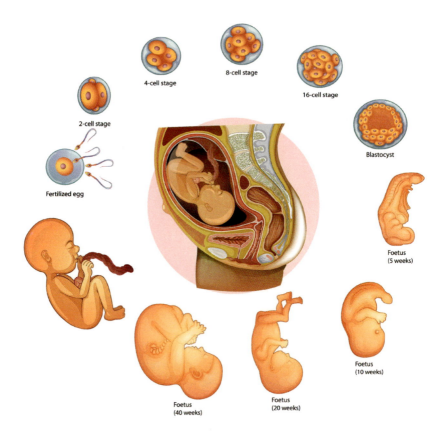

Fig. 4.4. Stages of the intrauterine development of a baby

soul! Here are the stages of development of a baby that are not taught in medical schools.

First month: The construction of very delicate cells into an entire body starts, and no one knows at this point if the baby will be female or male.

Second month: The fetus acquires its form, which will develop as either a boy or a girl. A male fetus has the shape of a globe, and a female fetus is shaped like a disk.

Third month: The five elements from which everything is comprised appear in the form of legs, arms, head, and body; at this point we know the sex of the baby.

Fourth month: This time signals the beginning of the crucial second trimester. At this point a baby girl already has all her eggs, gifted to her by her mother. The baby has formed limbs, head, and trunk, and it is possible to distinguish a boy from a girl. The baby has completed the formation of its heart, and the mother can feel its impulses and desires. She is not guided by her own preferences and tastes, but rather by the needs of the child, especially the child's need to also connect with its father. This month is called the month of two hearts (or rather three hearts, including that of the father).

Fifth month: This is the month of the flesh and blood waking up from hibernation. The baby's mind awakens, and spiritual qualities form. Bone marrow appears, and the skeletal, blood, and lymphatic systems are finally complete. The skin becomes elastic, covered with a lubricant rich in vitamins that protects the upper epithelium from exposure to water and keeps the nose, ears, and eyes from contact with the liquid inside.

Sixth month: This is the awakening of reason. The baby is capable of thinking. The formation of ligaments, joints, and hair completes during this time.

Seventh month: The formation of the physical body of the child is complete, and the formation of its subtle bodies and energy channels is underway.

Eighth month: This is the second most important month of the last trimester for the union of the mother and the child. It is the eighth month in standard calendar time, but it is actually the ninth lunar month. The spiritual bodies of mother and child prepare for the pending birth together. Closer to the tenth lunar month (or ninth calendar month), the child comes into tangible contact with both parents.

Ninth month: This is when all the sense organs, the mind, and the subtle bodies are ready to move from the mother's womb to the earthly space of love as intended by nature. The child is actively moving, pushing with its arms and legs. We observe bulges on the belly. The baby often hiccups, and the head begins to push the

104 Pregnancy

bones of the pelvis of the mother. The woman, anticipating what is to come, becomes physically and emotionally a dual system with her child. In childbirth they become a single unit. The job of the mother's secretion glands is to simultaneously signal both of the adrenal glands at the beginning of the birth phase. This is also when, to achieve a beautiful natural birth, the woman must develop a hormonal bouquet consisting of oxytocin and prostaglandins (accumulated in the umbilical cord of the baby), which stimulate love.

The sequence of delivery of all the other hormones during birth depends on the timeliness of the release of oxytocin, its quantity and quality, which depends on the mother's thoughts, actions, and feelings. Colostrum appears in the third month and starts building the nutrient properties of breast milk. A woman who does not devote all her precious attention to nurturing the child in her womb will not create enough colostrum, and later milk, which is vital for maintaining the health of the baby. It is thus very important for a woman to understand her own role in the formation of all the vital functions of the tiny human whom she bears, gives birth to, and nurtures, as well as the emotional climate of the family and the warmth of her husband's heart. The caring of her own parents and any older children or nephews and nieces, and even friends (in an unobtrusive way), can favorably affect the mother and the baby. In many cultures, the first weeks after birth are considered sacred in anchoring a child's soul in this world. It is not desirable to receive guests and arrange sumptuous celebrations during this precious time. The bonding of mother and child after the child has just landed and taken root on this planet is solidified during this time, so it is advisable for mother and child to take walks and dream together. Do not go shopping and do not put your child on display, no matter how proud you are of your wonderful offspring. Home births are especially sacred, and their intimacy should not be destroyed by the evaluative actions of doctors, masseurs, and breast-feeding "specialists" who did not participate in the bearing and birth of the child. Be patient; meditate more, engage in simple yoga with the baby, and receive and give massages in the family circle, which helps further the bond with the father of the family as well.

Water rituals are very important; daily ablutions with the baby will instill the instincts of swimming and diving. Everything the mother does in pregnancy is imprinted on the cellular and tactile levels of the baby, especially as the baby's abilities to hear, see, and empathize develop. Therefore we highly recommend when possible doing the Inner Smile (see chapter 2) and Six Healing Sounds (this chapter) meditations before conception, visualizing and structuring not only the body shell of the incoming soul, but also the positive gene matrix of the parents created by good thoughts, which effect positive qualities in the child on a cellular level. If the child was not planned for, then it is very worthwhile to recite positive affirmations that transform the memory of "mistakes" and change the experience that served as the beginning of the creation of new life. Here are some examples:

Through doubt, I found a mentor and expanded consciousness with new knowledge.
Now I understand responsibility.
I'm mature enough to continue my family line.
Pregnancy made my life crucial to a tiny human; this child is a continuation of me, and its future depends on my qualities.
I accept all changes in life as great gifts.
This child helped my heart open to love.

We believe that the information about our own intrauterine life as well as that of our children can help us deepen and expand our knowledge about our purpose and the sacredness of our path. From the very beginning, the egg is fertilized by the sperm. The first cell of a new organism, the zygote, is genetically identical to the human body. Embryologists say that between eighteen and twenty days after conception (three to four weeks of pregnancy), the baby's heart starts beating. By the twentieth day, the foundations of the nervous system are already forming. After five-and-a-half weeks, the baby starts moving its head.

106 Pregnancy

At six weeks, the baby can already move its entire body just like any adult, and at that point it is only four to five millimeters in length. The pregnant woman will only feel movement much later, at sixteen to twenty weeks. Mothers who have had many children feel the presence and movement of the baby earlier than that, however. If the baby was desired and the mother interacts with it not only on a subtle spiritual level but also by constantly stroking her belly, smiling, singing, listening to music, and eating food, this makes these mutually enjoyable experiences for both the expectant mother and the child. Likewise, a man who supports his partner in mutual parenthood not only becomes more humane as a person but also increases his creative potential.

Back in the 1990s in England, a scanner was invented that allowed you to see in color how an eight-week-old baby, whose face is the size of a strawberry, yawns, smiles, and cries. Remember the hero Aureliano, who shook the world in the novel *One Hundred Years of Solitude* by Gabriel Garcia Marquez, because he cried loudly while still in his mother's womb? Then it was perceived as an impossible metaphor,* but now we know more about life on Mother Earth, its tragedies and triumphs. At nine to ten weeks, a child starts moving its eyeballs, knows how to swallow, moves its tongue, hiccups, and alternates between states of wakefulness and sleep.

Starting at about eleven weeks, the baby begins to suck its thumb as part of the preparation for future sucking and to get microdoses of oxygen with a little water. The baby responds to sounds, and at this point external noises can wake it up. At the same time, tiny hands and feet are formed, including fingernails. During the sixteenth week eyelashes appear.

Many of these intrauterine impressions remain in our subconscious for life. Three great scholars, Stanislav Grof, Leonard Orr, and Jim Leonard, masters of transpersonal psychology, found the keys to

---

*Silent and withdrawn, Aureliano "weeps" in his mother's womb. His eyes are open at birth. Clairvoyant, he is possessed of prophetic powers. Readers of the novel are inclined to relate his prophetic talent to his having wept in his mother's womb.

transforming our original negative matrices into positive experiences through cyclic breathing, a form of breathing peculiar to the newborn immediately after entering into the air environment. This has allowed a huge number of adults to go through the process of their conception and birth once again, the purpose being to get rid of the painful imprinting of their uselessness and insecurity in their relationships with their parents and the personal traumas they experienced in the medical birthing model, and to in a sense be "reborn" in their original, natural state of trust and love.

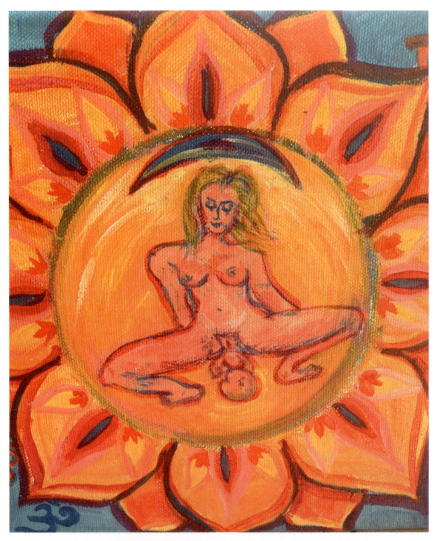

Illustration by Marina Dadasheva-Drown

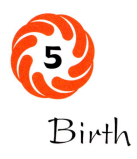

Birth

As birth approaches, the child recognizes its mother's feelings and reactions when exposed to harmonious or disharmonious situations and influences, especially sounds. Closer to birth the child has less room to move around, so it listens more, processing information that penetrates the womb from the outside that is imprinted in the mother's thoughts and reactions to that information. That is why by this time the expectant mother's body begins to actively produce the antistress hormones, which do not dull her maternal instincts but rather help her draw her gaze inward, deep into herself. At this time the woman should refrain from social interactions, and if she has a job she should take a leave of absence. It is also very helpful to bring expectant mothers together in groups, not so much to prepare for childbirth as to get support for conscious and responsible motherhood, for the health and life of the child depends on their mothering skills.

Expectant mothers must realize how sensitive the being they carry within them is and should live in a smile and in love. Do not be afraid to express your joy—laugh loudly and lovingly from the heart. This joy will transfer to your child, as all the cells of your body and mind will be vibrating with creative life force to prepare for childbirth.

TIMING

The timing of the birth of the baby depends on the temperament of the mother and the impulses of the baby, as well as the lunar phase. A 2020 study by Japanese scientists concluded:

> the findings . . . are consistent with the hypothesis [that] natural nighttime parturition is influenced by lunar phase, particularly the full moon, and thus they are consistent with the belief [that] the moon exerts an affect upon the timing of human birth. We speculate [that] the long-held belief [in] the association between birth and lunar phase may be based on historical observations that in the absence of artificial light at night, nocturnal births occurred in elevated number when the full moon brightly illuminated the nighttime sky.[1]

Nature can exert an influence on timing in other ways as well, as recalled in the following anecdote.

Marina's Field Notes

When I gave birth to my first child, nature was raging with an unusually strong blizzard. The cold intensified my movements, and I was happy to see the first snow and began to build a snowman just as the first inklings of the birth process signaled me that the time was coming soon. My labor lasted only forty-five minutes. Although the birth took place in a hospital, the baby was born right into my arms while I was in a squatting position. This was surprising and unusual for the time, 1972. My next child was born during a summer thunderstorm in 1976. My other children also chose active lunar-solar phases and the loud presence of nature. Later I began to take special note of the help that nature provided in the births of my grandchildren. The children of my eldest son were met by rosy dawns following storms in May and November. Crystal sparkles were dripping from wet leaves, and the birds were singing into the open window. The two babies of my eldest daughter were both born during evening storms during which the sky was ablaze with lightning, and the sounds of thunder merged with the song of my daughter's labor pains. My grandson and granddaughter were both born very quickly, in just two hours, thanks to nature's help.

It is crucial that parents recognize and honor nature and allow the child to feel its effects in the uterus during pregnancy as well as during birth. Each week is full of unique imprints of what the mother sees, hears, and does. The seven-month period is very significant for a baby as it brings the ability to hear, followed shortly thereafter by the ability to see with the inner eye and recognize colors. This is the result of the production of DNA methylation, which protects the baby from the stresses that occur during the last months of pregnancy, as the baby is big and its "house" has become small, so it has less room to move around. As well, the baby's need for light and sound increases because the external environment is shaping and structuring its genes. Just before birth, the baby starts micro-breathing, since the water in the womb contains oxygen. The mother should nest at home in preparation for the sacrament of birth by doing yoga, Chi Kung, and plunging into water and holding her breath for as long as possible, which prevents hypoxia or asphyxia, which can happen during childbirth.

BIRTHING POSITION AND ENVIRONMENT

The effects of all of the mother's activities are transmitted to the baby. Rhythmic breathing during birth affects the psychomotor system of the newborn and jumpstarts the activity of the baby's kidneys and liver, crucial organs that perform more than five hundred functions.

The state of health and the adaptive functions of the baby's body that help it acclimate to its new environment depend on the position in which the mother gives birth. In the last stage of childbirth—the "expulsion of the fetus" in the medical system's stark terms—adrenaline plays an important role. At this point if the mother has the instinct to assume a vertical position, this is natural for childbirth and also is the best position for breast-feeding, as the newborn hears its mother's heartbeat and presses against her stomach for the speedy delivery of the placenta following the birth. This position also protects the baby from the outside world.

The moment of transition from the aquatic environment of the womb into a space filled with air can be made smoother and more harmonious for the emerging human if the birth takes place in water, which allows the mother to be more comfortable and contributes to the easy separation of the placenta. The baby begins to suckle in the first few minutes, and the nutrient-dense placental blood slowly pours into the body of a newborn, enriching its immune system with stem cells and prostaglandins.

All the processes that began with conception continue through the natural birth process, up to and including the production of breast milk. The hormone oxytocin that stimulates the posterior lobe of the pituitary gland plays an active role not only in copulation and conception, but also in childbirth and lactation, justifying its being called the "creator of love." Oxytocin is directly related to the sex hormones testosterone and estrogen; it increases libido, provokes uterine contractions during orgasm, childbirth, and the separation of the placenta, and aids lactation. During the birthing process there's a whole supplementary bouquet that blossoms around oxytocin, the hormone of love; these are the morphine endorphins, which appear both in the mother and the child, fortifying their bond.

THE VITAL IMPORTANCE OF THE PLACENTA

Since ancient times, women who gave birth would chew on the placenta after the first breast-feeding session, thereby receiving a sufficient amount of prostaglandins through the saliva, which restores the body of the mother and strengthens her connection with the newborn. Nearly all mammals eat the placenta following birth.[2] The mother cuts off or takes a piece of the placenta from the birth assistant, holds it in her mouth behind a cheek, and then washes it down with an herbal infusion and a small amount of red wine for the fastest absorption of the placenta's stem cells into her blood. This ritual of health is now widely promoted in midwifery circles.

Multidisciplinary studies have been conducted on the positive effect that placental stem cells have on the immunization of a human and on preventing or eliminating any predisposition for genetic diseases in the family lineage.[3] Our long experience confirms the validity of this panacea. The physical and emotional health that is established during the perinatal and postnatal periods via the placenta helps immunize the child against what in medical parlance is called "the legacy of distorted love."[4] This is commonly the result of narcissistic parents failing to imprint a child with parental love during all phases of conception, pregnancy, and birth, as well as during the perinatal period. Even a traumatic condition such as autism can be attributed to this "distortion." The lack of an ability to love is most likely imprinted on the chromosomes of one or both of the parents and transmits to the child in a repeat of the family legacy of narcissism—something that may be difficult for the person with an undistorted program of love imprinting to understand. And no matter how much you try to impress such concepts as compassion and sensitivity on people with a more developed reptilian part of their brain, they will not understand what you're talking about, as the problem starts before birth. Love for one's own comfort and the desire to control others—the traits of narcissism—are not the results of one's upbringing, but rather the result of something that started even before birth.

Given the vital function of the placenta, it is important that it not be separated from the umbilical cord due to its nutritional value and preventative functions. The umbilical cord very quickly becomes dry yet flexible, and firm enough to be snapped. Nature itself will show you when it's time for the umbilical cord to fall off of the umbilical ring. Allowing this to happen naturally will prevent the possibility of a stress-induced umbilical hernia. In the past in Russia as well as in other parts of the world, the placenta was considered an incarnation of the guardian angel of the child. People would perform ceremonies urging the angel to protect the newborn from the evil eye and evil forces. If the child was born with a lifeless, thin umbilical cord, then perhaps it provided insufficient nourishment and protection for the child. If the baby comes out weak or lifeless but the umbilical cord has not broken off immediately after birth, there are more chances to bring the child back to life. In cases where the umbilical cord is strong and so is the placenta, resuscitation is performed through massage of the placenta and simultaneous taps on the child's spine (baby yoga).

THE PERINATAL PERIOD

The first day is a very important time for engaging the spiritual and emotional bodies of the child, on which the development of its physical body depends. If the delivery has been difficult, it's best to put the baby in a warm bath from time to time and pour some cold water on the crown of its head to boost the child's immune system; this is best done by the mother. It helps the baby's circulation and energizes the channels along and inside the spine that comprise the Microcosmic Orbit, stabilizing the neuroendocrine, chakra, and acupressure systems.

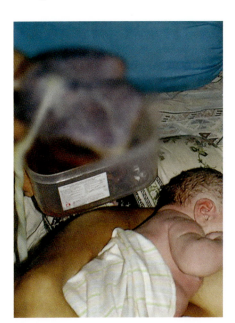

Fig. 5.1. Placenta with the umbilical cord attached

Thumb-sucking has a positive effect on the psyche of the child and helps it cope with the echoes of its birth trauma in the perinatal period. Such trauma can occur when labor has been induced or when there has been an episiotomy, C-section, or premature cutting of the umbilical cord before its pulsation has stopped. Emotional trauma can occur due to the separation of the child from its mother in the first minutes and hours of life. It happens quite often in medical settings that the baby is not immediately presented to the mother's breast—not even within the first half hour—which deprives the baby of the final stage of birth: sucking and tasting the precious elixir of life, the colostrum-enriched breast milk, which is a guarantee of lifelong immunity and a high level of vitamins and the hormones of love and immunoglobulin. Colostrum is commonly used in medicine for its strong antibody factors (usually it ends up losing its original pristine quality). Its nutritional profile is immediate, so the earlier the breast is offered, the better for the baby.

Sometimes in medical settings babies are not given to their mothers for several days after birth. This damages the bonding process and lowers the natural maternal instinct in women. For several decades now there has been a previously unprecedented dispute between renowned doctors about how traumatic it is for a child to not get enough placental and umbilical cord blood immediately after birth. Doctoral dissertations have been defended and books written about this subject. Some of the first geneticists who proved the importance of not cutting the umbilical cord were even imprisoned for making such a claim. Since the 1990s, no one in the medical system seems to be interested in making sure that the baby gets this blood. The common hospital rules are deceitful and do not allow the child to receive its health benefit due to the practice of clamping the umbilical cord with a special clip, which does not allow a drop of blood to pass from the placenta to the baby.

Moreover, the clamps are placed in two or even three spots along the length of the umbilical cord so that blood does not flow from the placenta. This blood, as well as colostrum, so rich in stem cells, gamma globulins, and prostaglandins, is wasted, and in some circumstances

116 Birth

becomes a donor substance. Very few mothers are allowed to learn about the fate of their placenta and the roughly 100 grams of additional "best blood" that you or your baby were deprived of. And this might be okay if the genetic parental codes did not register in so many babies at the level of anemia, and sometimes even asphyxia, since breathing is stimulated by blood flow. After a baby is separated from its familiar home in the womb, so generous in nutrition, it can be subjected to unfriendly bacteria while in a state of reduced immunity. This is especially common when at birth the baby is taken away from its mother and her friendly bacteria and her loving arms, which bring security and trust.

Marina's Field Notes

One boy, freeborn in a Lotus Birth in the sea, escaped the genetic disease on his father's side, epilepsy, inherent in all males in the family. The umbilical cord was kept for three days, and on the fourth it fell from the closed umbilical ring of the child by itself. Every day the baby dived and swam with his parents in the ocean waters with the placenta, and after the swimming sessions, the placenta was salted and stored in a "breathing" container—a box with holes. A few months later, the parents and the baby returned to their life as a typical Japanese family and went on to have two more sons, who did not have a Lotus Birth and have both inherited the genetic disease of epilepsy from the father's side of the family. The parents were very upset that they did not birth these kids at home or in the sea, and so the next time they gave birth to their baby in a country house and in bathwater. Their daughter was born a perfectly healthy girl, and not long afterward her older brothers, having spent time with her and thanks to the motivation of their parents, received the potential of health and almost got a new code of imprints.

My eldest son, who was born right into my arms, although in the hospital, managed to avoid the kind of quick separation from the placenta usually imposed by the medical system due to my vigorously insisting that the cord not be cut. The navel was tied only after the placenta was delivered, and we thereby avoided the disease of diabetes, hereditary on his father's side, which ended up being transferred to the children of my husband's siblings.

A soft separation of the placenta from the uterus occurs naturally if the child remains on the umbilical cord. In this case, the woman avoids possible bleeding caused by a sharp detachment, which happens when the blood from the umbilical cord suddenly rushes back to the placenta and not the other way around, as is natural.

Many women know that substances made from placentas (usually animal) make the best and most useful makeup, as it restores a beautiful, youthful complexion. Human and animal placentas are also routinely used in other consumer products, including pharmaceuticals, hair-care products, and health tonics and foods. Human placentas and umbilical cords are also used in stem cell transplantation.

The best and most natural thing to do is to return the blood to the child, who during the very challenging sacrament of birth—squeezing through a narrow birth canal and having its body pressed in the process—drops a portion of its blood back into the placenta so that this valuable elixir can be returned to the baby after birth.

CORD-CUTTING

The paradox of birthing children in hospitals, ostensibly to provide a safe environment that protects the health of mother and child, is that less and less time is given to the placenta and the umbilical cord for their postpartum benefits for the newborn. Within about ten seconds following birth, the clamps are brought out and cutting rapidly occurs. You can ask to have your baby placed on your belly with the umbilical cord still attached, but they'll still clamp it. That is why every woman should learn about the vital significance and mission of the placenta.

The umbilical cord contains two thick-walled arteries and one thin-walled vein. Blood flows through the vein from the placenta to

118 Birth

the baby, and venous blood flows through the arteries in the opposite direction. Blood circulation is supported by the heartbeat of the mother to the intrauterine baby. The baby in turn pumps the blood through the entire length of the umbilical cord, ensuring its smooth return. It is absolutely clear that there is no time limit allotted for the pulsation of the umbilical cord and the continuous return of blood to the baby, a process designed by nature in the perinatal period.

Marina's Field Notes

What I am about to describe is not surprising in the course of the natural birth of a baby who was not subjected to the medical system. A wonderful couple was anticipating their first baby together (each of the spouses already had two grown children from previous relationships), conceived in love and in the desire to give birth in a state of love and in nature. They came by train from Russia through Manchuria and China to our home in Thailand. From the very beginning of the pregnancy they had attended natural birth groups and had said no to any interventions to natural birth. That meant that ultrasounds and plane flights were completely out of the question. I was a little worried about their weeklong train ride, but the child's mother was very centered, and the father supported her and the baby in all her reasonable and well-informed decisions. By the way, the woman had a medical background, but this did not deter her from eschewing the medical approach to the birth process. The couple were already practicing Healing Love and Tantra, were aware of the importance of erogenous zones in childbirth, and had mastered the skill of opening the secret gates.

In working with them I learned more about loving creativity in a couple. Obviously, the not very successful experiences they'd each had in their first marriages had led the couple to a path of wisdom in their new family relationship. They decided on freebirth for their first child together. In her previous pregnancy the woman had a separated pubic symphysis after the delivery, which required a long recovery. Possibly that is why during this pregnancy her baby, at just a little over two pounds, decided to be born one month before term. The birth was truly beautiful—quite fast, orgasmic, and ending in an unexpected conclusion.

During the birth, the water in the bath remained completely transparent, and even after the birth of the beautiful, smiling baby, the tub was absolutely clean, and the umbilical cord was very strong, thick, and a healthy pinkish-purple color. It pulsed with a soft flow of blood for two hours while the mother and her newborn stayed in the water and felt great. When the woman decided to get out of the bath, the pulsation slowed down but did not stop. The placenta, entirely whole and healthy, maybe just slightly pale from the decrease in pulsations, was delivered almost five hours later after the baby. The parents completed the ritual of the Lotus Birth by giving the placenta to the earth and planting a wonderful palm tree over it with a prayer and a celebratory meal for the guests. In the evening, a ritual fire was lit in honor of the placenta while rice paper balloons were launched into the sky. Everyone was happy with the completion of the placental ritual. The baby girl grew and developed very actively, enjoying cold water showers, swimming in the lake, in waterfalls, and in the pool.

Not long after this experience, a couple of musicians awaiting their firstborn arrived at my door. The mother had received abdominal surgery during her student years in the United States; she also arrived with a medical warning about the weakness of her body and the recommendation that she should have a cesarean section. At almost the same time another wonderful mother was about to have her second freebirth, water-born child. She was a yoga instructor, and the baby's birth happened so fast that they barely had enough time to fill the bathtub. I guided them through a video call. Actively pulsing, the placenta was born a few minutes after the baby, and I could practically feel the pulsation of the placenta over the computer for quite some time after the birth. It continued to infuse the little princess with healing blood nectar along with a nourishing river of grace in the form of colostrum.

The musician couple had meanwhile decided to birth their baby in the beautiful villa of our friends, where there was a bath and a large

120 Birth

inflatable pool. The father played the violin, and the mother sang through her contractions. The boy was born in a tantric embrace pose to the kisses of his parents. Mother and baby, completely healthy, spent an hour expecting the birth of the pulsating umbilical cord. The baby grew pinker in color, and the placenta was delivered easily, already pale with blue clots and residual blood. We usually place the placenta in a beautiful vessel where it is examined and washed and bring it along for each swimming and bathing session with the child.

Five days later, a wonderful placental feast took place for the two couples and their little heroes, and now trees grow in the luxurious alley of flowers and bushes where the placentas were eventually buried.

Not long afterward came another truly wonderful pool birth, in the middle of a garden surrounded by rosebushes. This was the birth of another little princess who decided to come out of her mom (a beautiful and smart woman) buttocks-first, conventionally known as a breech birth. This baby was born when her mother was almost thirty-six years old, her first child. The father of the child was present during the birth and was tremulous and obedient, a loving disciple of his queen. The couple lived in different countries, so their coming together for the momentous occasion of the delivery of the baby was a tantric melody, a multi-orgasmic fairy tale of their love made manifest. Why the girl decided to be born in the breech position remains a mystery, only the baby knows the answer, and the parents can only guess. Three days after the birth, the beautiful placental ritual was performed, which the parents had been dreaming about even during the pregnancy.

One evening we received an urgent phone call from some friends who asked us to help a young couple who'd given birth at home that morning, but the placenta had not been delivered yet. The couple refused to go to the hospital: "We didn't choose home birth to end up in the hospital" was their attitude. The danger of possible infection that could occur if the detached placenta remained in the uterus for too long did not phase them. When I arrived, the screaming baby was lying on the mother's belly, and the father was helplessly fussing around them. The baby had not yet been taken to the breast and the parents did not know how to help her. As soon as we properly attached the baby to the breast she latched on and started sucking with great appetite. The young mother felt contractions coming on, and standing in a Chi Kung position with the nursing baby in her arms she delivered the placenta. After processing and washing the birth canal, I explained that I needed money to pay for a taxi. The couple happily reported that they didn't have any money and that the call to me was just a plea for help. I explained to them the measure of their and my own responsibility for the health of the mother and the baby; they replied that they would take care of this on their own. I had no choice but to leave them with necessary herbs and things to care for the baby and mother; they even asked me for money for food before I left.

This shows that the work of assistants in childbirth is not easy and, as it turns out, should be selfless. Another case: again, a very young girl and her rather irresponsible older partner gave birth to a baby, and I was informed by telephone that the placenta had already come out but would not separate. I asked them to call for medical help, but I understood that there was no time to spare. My fears were confirmed: after the birth of the child, the young, inexperienced father began to press on the mother's belly, knowing that she had to deliver the remaining part without realizing its physiological purpose in the first minutes and hours of the perinatal period. With remarkable strength he pulled down on the entire peritoneum, and a part of the uterus ended up at the entrance to the vagina. Thankfully, his actions didn't cause bleeding, and the uterus with the partially separated placenta was gently returned to its place. After what could have been a disaster, and with the help of a soft, noninvasive contact massage along with buzzing sound vibrations, the placenta finally left the woman's body.

These are examples of how self-confidence and intuition take precedence over science. Thirty years ago, in many countries around the world, because of hospital rules about assisting in childbirth and the insistence on cutting the umbilical cord right away as well as the practice of

122 Birth

separating babies from their mothers, home birth has gained in popularity. Traditional birthing practices do not always conveniently fit into modern clinical obstetrics care, which is why more frequently now couples want home births in water or ocean births, thanks to the pioneering work of people like Michel Odent, Ina May Gaskin, and Chris Griscom.

AFTER-BIRTH CARE

Following natural birth it is necessary to treat the birth canal with propolis, massage, and herbal infusions. Strengthening exercises for the peritoneum and sex organs should also be included in after-birth care for the mother. After the blood secretions cease, Taoist practice recommends training sessions with a jade egg as well as Ovarian Breathing (for both exercises, see chapter 1) and constant massage of the breasts ("Warming the Breasts," see chapter 1), with the gradual introduction of Chi Kung exercises and yoga asanas. Inverted poses and bridge pose are very useful. For the spine and back we recommend Tao Yin Yoga practice ending with the Six Healing Sounds meditation found in chapter 4. Both should be done in a chair (chair yoga) or lying on your back, which is especially recommended after a rapid delivery and prolonged labor. In many cultures where friends and relatives assist in childbirth, there are ceremonies of closing the birth, which helps regenerate the mother and ground the baby, whose body is vulnerable to interference by medical professionals who are strangers.

Water has a great influence on the gentle transition of the child from the womb to the air environment, especially while the umbilical cord still pulsates. At this time it is advisable to pour warm water over the baby's head. Its body can be very gently washed, aiming a stream of water in an infinity shape, all the while supporting the baby under its head in a water-filled tub. If there is mucus in the respiratory tract as indicated if the baby wheezes and does not suck on the nipple even twenty minutes after birth, very soft underwater dives can help, as they will water down and push out the mucus. This is something that parents need to learn from their experienced birth assistant ahead of time, but the assistant should still partake in these kinds of rehabilitation processes. For children with tight or multiple umbilical cord entanglements, a water birth in a squatting position is safer than lying on your back or sitting in a chair; this way the transition from the aquatic environment of the womb into the same water environment will not cause the cord to tighten around the neck and makes it easier to remove the cord in the water. There is more time for bonding in the water, too, eye-to-eye and skin-to-skin. The blood from the placenta to the baby will shimmer with good emotional information, and the bonding is secured for the following years up until puberty, and sometimes even for the rest of the mother and child's lives.

The second panacea of absolute health after the placental blood is the maternal colostrum meal received by the baby immediately after birth, accompanied by the sucking reflex that is so necessary for brain development. Colostrum helps the child engage its motor skills, allowing the baby to more easily learn to crawl, stand up, and hold her breath under water. Colostrum is very important not only because of the protein content (casein, which breaks down differently in adult bodies), carbohydrates (in the form of lactose), and fat (in the form of lipids), but also because it has a significant immunobiological effect. Colostrum contains complex proteins and natural antibodies that bind foreign substances (antigens) that the newly born organism might come into contact with. In addition, this original milk contains physiological antibiotics that can counteract possible sepsis, intestinal diseases, and pneumonia. Hypogalactia, or low milk supply, is a disease provoked by late application to the breast; the condition deprives the baby not only of necessary nutrients, but also natural immunization.

In childbirth, a woman must be guided by her instincts, not her head. It is important to understand this even before conception, and maybe even before the start of the partnership. Sexuality should flow in the right direction, with consideration for the personal health of the future mother and child rather than mindlessly satisfying curious sexual appetites. A woman's health is the health of her child and the continuation

124　Birth

of a strong family tree. Modern society pulls a woman away from her instincts to give birth in a quiet, secluded place, without bright lights, in complete intimacy. Let's not repeat the mistakes of the past; let's allow our instincts to kick in. It all begins with the fact that in giving birth, a woman needs to be with her baby, feed and caress her, teaching her baby everything she knows. Will she choose cold-water hardening, or immunization through vaccination? Will she help her baby adapt to temperature changes by dousing with cold water and allowing for active movements, or by swaddling, which prevents any movement and leads to lack of thermoregulation? Will she maintain immunity by frequent breast-feeding sessions and loving touch, or with synthetic vitamin pills? These are the choices: head or heart, fear or trust.

The chromosomes of the child capture not only the physiological information of the parents, but also the mood of the parents. All the foundations of a newborn's emotional health are established prenatally and perinatally. In fact, everything that happens to the mother becomes the baby's first learning matrix. If the mother is well-prepared for the birth, the baby is also thoroughly prepared for it. Diving and swimming with breath-holding will help the infant to not panic if suddenly there is a shortage of oxygen. Active movements and yoga, which are necessary for the mother during pregnancy, also create a matrix for the baby to learn how to move in the world by rounding its body, pushing, and turning its head and shoulders. If the mother is optimistic and knows what she needs for a harmonious natural birth, the in-utero child will read this information, and everything will turn out perfectly on a level of trust. If the mother dives during pregnancy and childbirth, the child will know how to dive as soon as it's born. After birth, gently guiding the child from the head and diving, singing soothing and relaxing melodies, and pouring water over the baby's head will ensure that the baby will not experience fear after moving from the water element of the womb to the air environment. This baby is not going to fear water and will gladly dive and swim with her parents, and later with friends.

If the child is not subjected to medical interventions and hospitals and swaddling immediately after birth, this child will strengthen its respiratory, muscular, and cerebral abilities. A baby still in an embryonic state can breathe underwater by micro-breathing, since water contains oxygen. With every minute of its development, the fetus becomes more and more human. It moves, somersaults, sucks its thumb, pulls at the umbilical cord, smiles and cries, overcomes the difficulties of moving through the birth canal, spreads the maternal bones, screws itself into the birth canal, presses, pushes, and finally is born! A tiny human has made it and can now look forward to becoming a creative human being with limitless possibilities.

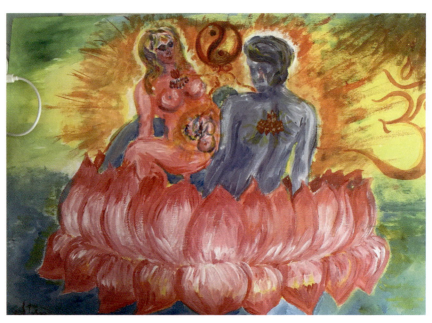

Illustration by Marina Dadasheva-Drown

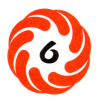

Family Care

Having given birth to a healthy baby, a woman continues to co-create with her partner, teaching him how to interact with the child and the natural elements as she nurtures the balance between yin and yang energies. An active lifestyle that includes the father in activities such as yoga, swimming, and sports expands the father's bonding with the child. The father's playfulness with the baby, throwing the child up in the air as if flying, brings smiles and laughter. The baby learns to have fun engaging his bone and muscle systems, and then completely relaxes in the strong arms that hold him with such tenderness. The father teaches the baby to be active; the mother nourishes and instills a healthy lifestyle. The first seconds of earthly breathing are what give us the strongest pattern for life here on planet Earth.

Both parents must be involved in this life-awakening process. There must be no disagreements, sleepless nights, and interventions from grandparents. In the first days and weeks following the birth of a child it is very important that the parents are inspired by the intimacy of their family life, and so they should try to embrace this blessed event without seeking assistance from the outside world. Keeping the baby on the tummy (the mother's or the father's) contributes to the baby's instinct to crawl. Daily contact with water in a large bath or pool is a continuation of the security of the womb, allowing the baby to exercise and be unafraid of water.

128   Family Care

The Inner Smile (see chapter 2) and Six Healing Sounds (see chapter 4) are fundamental practices of the Universal Healing Tao, the roots of the great Tree of Life. The trunk, with its deep and powerful roots, is strengthened by the physical practices of Chi Kung, Tai Chi, Tao Yin Yoga, and other Taoist trainings that develop and balance the harmony of yin and yang in the body. To create flexible branches with luxuriant foliage, nourishment in the form of increasing and balancing the energy potential of all the elements is required. The basic practices of Taoist Healing Love nurture the luxurious crown of the tree, uniting the person with Heaven and Earth. By practicing these ceremonies of purification and filling our bodies with the great energy of chi, we become one with the multi-orgasmic universe, which allows the tree to blossom. The highest transformation occurs with a third fundamental Taoist practice, the Microcosmic Orbit (see chapter 2), which cultivates the immortality of the soul and the long life of the body.

Any form of exercise that appeals to you will strengthen muscles that have been stretched during pregnancy. Breathing practices contribute to diaphragmatic mobility, stimulating the organs. Working in the garden with a shovel and a hoe is a very simple and practical way to maintain the shape of your breasts. Best of all are the exercises of Chi Kung, which can be combined with yoga asanas to fully restore the body of the mother after pregnancy and childbirth. Besides helping a woman recover from pregnancy, these practices harmonize the emotional climate of the family and encourage the involvement of the father in the upbringing of the baby.

THE MOTHER MATRIX

Recently a video came out—it was only a few minutes long—about a mother who had died in childbirth and whose heart had been transplanted into a young man who would otherwise have died. It was later found that when woman's baby cried, even if compassionate, caring people tried to calm the baby down—grandmothers and mothers of other kids, fathers, teachers, and a nurse—the bitter crying continued.

Family Care   **129**

But when the young man who now had the heart of the baby's mother picked him up and held him close to his heart, the baby stopped crying and started smiling and touching and studying the man with his hands. The child's heart had picked up the vibrations of his mother's heart from the young man's field.

Joseph Chilton Pearce says that a child is affected by the family matrix through three natural imperatives: language, vision, and the intelligence of the heart. And all of these develop through the child's interaction with its parents. Of great importance is the period of breast-feeding because of the constant contact with the heart, face, and especially the eyes of the mother from the moment of birth to the twelfth week after it. Besides providing nutrition, breast-feeding stimulates a visual awareness of reality and an awakened consciousness, and further strengthens the maternal bond.

Not so long ago children grew up in families participating in all the activities of the home and the farm. As a result, they were friendly with the animal world, aware of the natural world, and had exceptional health and energy and an amazing ability to adapt to their environment. Nowadays the family matrix has been fractured by an educational system that is more interested in programming young minds than helping kids think for themselves; add to this the ubiquity of cell phones and addictive computer games, not to mention junk foods laden with poisons that have no nutritional value. Even young children suffer from allergies, and obesity is common, even in young children. How can a newborn feel love and trust if they've never known their mother's breast and were bottle-fed, injected with toxic vaccines, and fed junk food? But it is not impossible to have a course correction, as the following anecdote illustrates.

Marina's Field Notes

At one time we used to take into our family the most difficult children in the age group between four and six to spend a short time with us. We changed their diet and their activities. On Sundays we had

130 Family Care

family outings at a community pool. There we renewed eye contact with the children, and the joy of playing in the water together fortified our connection. During those sessions at the pool we also met with couples who were preparing to adopt, and we taught them how to swim together as a family and how to bond with kids who may have never experienced bonding.

An especially significant result was obtained in our work with a five-year-old boy who'd been diagnosed with autism and overfed with sweets and fried foods. The child loved hugging and smiled at every kind word. There were four kids in his family, and they had been left to their own devices in finding whatever care and love they could. This boy was the youngest in his family. At least he hadn't been given pharmaceutical drugs for his condition. During the day his parents worked on their farm, and evenings were spent with popcorn in front of the TV. As a result, the boy couldn't walk very well and had poor coordination due to being overweight.

We worked with the boy's parents and siblings to show a different way of living. After being exposed to the trampoline and the swimming pool and learning what it's like to have your older siblings read fairy tales to you at night, and how it feels to build Legos with your older brother, he quickly gained mobility and his speech normalized. Heartfelt kindness and expressions of love fixed the lost connection in the boy. After a year of unobtrusive work with the boy's whole family, the diagnosis of autism was removed. We practiced the Inner Smile with the parents and taught them soft contact massage. It took a year for the boy to achieve responsiveness.

Another interesting case involved a four-year-old boy with cerebral palsy who was unable to speak and had poor hearing. Fortunately, his parents were still madly in love, and they also knew the boy had special needs. To address his needs the family happily mastered basic Taoist meditations and daily Chi Kung practice, and the simplest form of Tai Chi. We began to train the family in the water, at home in the bath and in the community pool on weekends, so the boy could splash around and play and learn to hold his breath and not panic. The boy quickly

Family Care **131**

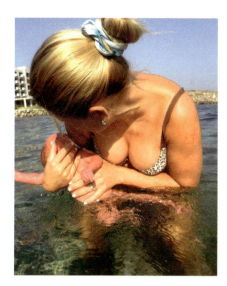

Fig. 6.1. Children learning to be at home in the water, jumping on a trampoline, and swimming in a pool

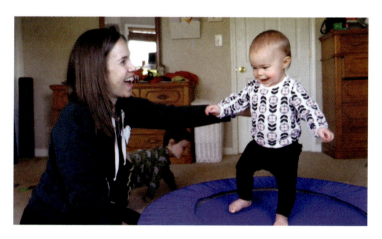

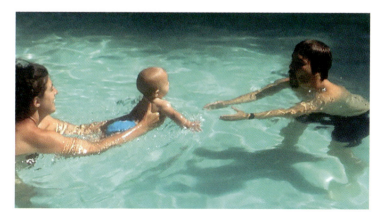

learned how to dive, and he would tumble and play with his newborn sister, so both children quickly learned how to swim. Two months later, the boy could stand on his feet and began to say his first word, "Dada," to his father. His progress inspired everyone who witnessed it, and by request we started classes on Chi Kung and Taoist yoga for a group of like-minded people.

Nowadays, people no longer raise large families, as this primal act of creation has lost its value in modern society. Michel Odent, described as "the doctor who encouraged women to experience pain-free labor in warm pools of water and was the first to write about the importance of placing newborn babies to the breast, has turned Cassandra. His new book is a warning to humanity that we face a grim future by our heedless embrace of medical technology; that the very techniques used to save lives are also changing the human race on an evolutionary level."[1] Odent now says, "Family has become a short-term phenomenon. In itself it is a nonviable and unnatural model of relations." Then he adds an unexpected clarification: "However, when the nuclear family is the nucleus of the extended family, and the extended family the nucleus of society, everything works beautifully. If we strip away the extended family, the nucleus explodes."

The family is governed by the maternal principle and spiritual sex. This is the basis of the mother matrix. Since ancient times, the mother has been the guardian of the home, giving birth to children and feeding them with her milk. A woman's instinct to feed and procreate is inherent in the ancient brain, helping to preserve not only her sexual desire but also her loyalty to the father of her children. A woman instinctively wishes to preserve a loving, joyful atmosphere in the family, and such a mother will always pass on to her children a good inheritance, not only chromosomal, but emotional and spiritual as well. Of course, the role of the father is undeniable. If one of the spouses puts the responsibility for the integrity of the family and the education of the children on the other, then what happens is

Family Care   133

that the father says, "If you changed, everything would be fine," or the mother says, "If you spent more time with the children, you would be a better father." This kind of manipulation destroys trust in the family and often leads to divorce and broken homes. Children who have been left to their own devices are among the unhappiest people in the world. They grow up to be unhappy with themselves and dissatisfied in their relationships with others.

The process of individuation starts around the time a child loses his baby teeth, around the age of six. A lot of interesting things about this can be gleaned from the books of Rudolf Steiner, the founder of Waldorf schools, which in the last century have reconciled religion, culture, and education to create a coherent image of a developing human being. Up until the first signs of puberty, a child's mental body is inseparable from that of her parents; she has no personal experience in relation to the state and to society. If the parents abdicate their responsibility and leave the child to her own devices during this time, there will be significant losses: as a teenager they will lack focus or they may enter the illusory world of drugs, not having any other way to adapt to life. What do we do in a situation like this?

Earlier we talked about the circle of creation and the interaction of the elements, the basis for the interdependence of all life. This Taoist principle points to the influence and dependence of every organ on all the others. We can create a circle of destruction or a beautiful and natural creation through our inner microcosm and the connection between the elements. Conflict is always present in our lives, but it can always be neutralized by positive intentions and actions. Here's what conflict in the elements, as seen in the destructive cycle of nature, looks like: Water extinguishes and suppresses the energy of fire, and its ability to burn wood and nourish the earth. Fire acts as the parent of earth. Earth is a child of water. Metal cuts and destroys wood. Wood is the parent of fire. Fire can destroy and melt metal. Earth blocks water. Water is the parent of wood. Wood can deenergize earth and drink all the water.

When we fill our lower tan tien cauldron, the goblet of energy

134 *Family Care*

at the center of the abdomen, with the energy of earth, water gets pushed out. Metal can open up a stream of water. Fire ignites, burning wood. If we harmonize the female and male elements and their qualities within ourselves, we harmonize our inner space with the outside space and create a field of virtue. To connect the microcosmos that is our body with the universe, it is necessary to accept the energy potential of the natural forces. In the Tao we use the symbol of the pakua, an octagonal figure of eight trigrams, to indicate that the five elements balance one another thanks to the rotation of the drops of yin and yang inside the octagon.

In each trigram there is a certain number of unbroken yang and broken yin lines, symbolizing the compression activity of yin and the expansion activity of yang. The trigrams have correspondences in astronomy, astrology, geography, geomancy, anatomy, the family, and elsewhere. The eight trigrams of the pakua correspond to the "eight forces" and the "eight extraordinary meridians" in the body. In Chinese medicine there are eight forces of nature that correspond to various organs and that rule the body. Meridians are channels in the body through which energy passes. The eight extraordinary meridians are among the most important energy pathways. This meridian system is nurtured by the eight planets and the eight related star essences.

Bhagwan Shree Rajneesh, known as Osho, was universally recognized but not universally understood. A brilliant educator, he expanded our knowledge of the nature of human beings. He felt that many people in today's world deny themselves their primary mission—for men to live as husbands and for women to live as wives. He believed the modern overemphasis on individuation to be the direct cause of broken family ties, which results in children growing up feeling lost and alone.

Fathers

From conception to pregnancy, pregnancy to birthing, and birthing to life itself, fathers are indispensable. Men do not carry a baby in the womb

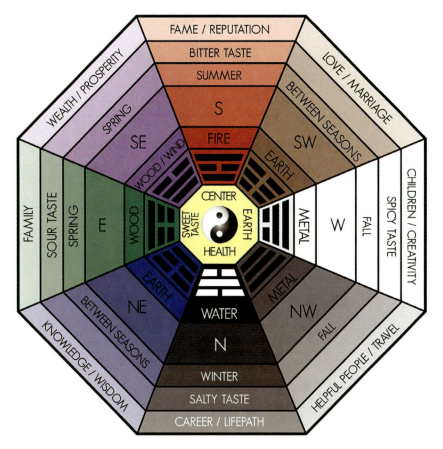

Fig. 6.2. Pakua Forming and Channel Opening

and therefore are less tactile with a newborn. Sometimes they do not even dare to take the baby in their arms, afraid to damage the tiny body, and so bonding does not happen. Taoist practice encourages the father's hands to be the first to receive the baby as it emerges, the excited father's heart beating in unison with the accomplishment of this miracle of life!

Stroking, massage, and sharing breast-feeding sessions invite the new father to participate in the process of building the baby's health. Conscious implementation of the father's imprinting and bonding will then happen for both parents.

Over twenty-five years ago, Colin Campbell Drown, who has

edited many books on the Universal Healing Tao, upon seeing for the first time a newborn baby in the hands of both of its parents, exclaimed, "Now the man is involved in the work of parenthood!" He went on to devote his life to this work, to become a father of many children as well as a grandfather, a spiritual obstetrician, and a trainer of children with disorders of the musculoskeletal and mental systems (autism, Down syndrome, and cerebral palsy). He has helped parents and children around the world with Taoist Healing Love and practices based on Chi Kung, Tai Chi, and yoga.

In these technological times, the bonding of both parents with the child has become particularly important. A breast-feeding woman shares a bond with her child, while all too often the man fades into the background to become only the provider of material things, and this is very damaging to his fatherhood. That is why the Universal Healing Tao emphasizes the role of the father in all aspects of conception, pregnancy, childbirth, and family care.

Talk to Your Children

Open, loving communication with your child is a guarantee that the child will become your soul mate and will follow you in all the family endeavors. It is especially good to make it clear to children that they are a source of love between Mom and Dad, and not a source of discord. Children are very responsive to parents who include them in all their expressions of love. For example, talk about the summer holidays, when Mom and Dad will be together and the kids can witness them kissing and hugging. Or talk about planning for a new baby or joyfully congratulate your young son or daughter on their growing up and having the right to their own space in the house. Children are ready to dream with their parents about moving to another city or to the country. Discuss with them the possibility of renovations to the house or planting trees, bushes, and flowers.

> ### 📝 Marina's Field Notes
>
> We met a beautiful young Canadian couple in a small town near Montreal who had given birth to two wonderful babies, a brother and a sister, two years apart, whom we trained in the methods of the Universal Healing Tao. The children had been born in multi-orgasmic love, but even more important, they were growing up in a family with loving parents who encouraged open communication and a creative, active lifestyle, traveling and experiencing adventures with their free-spirited grandparents. Even today, this couple still lives in great creativity and love. Their children are wonderful, gifted, respectful teenagers who do not boast about their many talents. Their main treasures are their kindness, a nonjudgmental view of life, and love for all living beings and plants. They are musical and social, and they travel the world with their parents, making movies, taking pictures, and painting.

One of the most important and significant moments in the life of a young child is when a dog or a cat comes along. Some children love birds and others are interested in amphibians. It is necessary to support this little caring person in their dream of having a pet to love and care for, even if at this time you cannot bring one into the home. Try to find an approach to the situation and don't cause unnecessary disappointment. Read books together about the new furry friend who will come into your home when you are ready to have a pet; slowly prepare its corner and begin to acquire what's necessary to care for a dog, a rabbit, or a bird. A child needs a friend to love and take care of; this teaches responsibility.

Even before pregnancy, decide on the changes in your life that will come after the birth of your child. Each person to a greater or lesser extent is inherently selfish; parents need to consciously work on this and not pass this on to their child.

138 Family Care

📝 Marina's Field Notes

I remember the elderly woman from whom we rented a summer house in the States. Our eight-month-old, freedom-loving baby loved to crawl between the beds of her garden and taste everything. He especially loved to pick tomatoes and dug up carrots directly from the ground. He dug up potatoes, tasted the cabbage, and later took interest in bell peppers. I apologized to our landlady and tried to limit his outings in the garden, but Mrs. Flanigan asked me not to stop my son, and she wholeheartedly supported his interest in vegetables. She would plant seeds with him at her side and teach him to weed the garden. She often told me how she raised her four sons and a daughter, and that now she often plays active games with her grandchildren near Lake Champlain, organizing various competitions in the water. Mrs. Flanigan's children had all moved to big cities but would visit her and her husband every summer break. She built separate summer houses for each of her children (like the one that we rented from her) so their activities would not disturb her husband, who was disabled. In the evenings she hosted dinners in their big, beautiful house. When our little ones joined them for dinner, the house immediately turned into a playground. I felt very nervous about this, but she always laughed. Her favorite phrase became a great support for me with my many children: "Every woman makes a decision; it is either a tidy house or children." She asked me not to worry because she and I had made the right choice.

And I know this for a fact: they say that children do not like vegetables, salads, and some fruits at an early age. I want to clarify—it all depends on how they get acquainted with them. If it happens directly in the garden, then the foundation of their friendship with vegetables is established. Now my baby is almost seventeen, and his favorite dish is salad! Whenever we go out to celebrate a family occasion, he orders a double portion of vegetables, everything green, with all the colors of the garden. The main thing is that I placed no restrictions on him trying and eating whatever he liked. Every child is smart, curious, free, and very sensitive before prohibitions come along. Keep it that way by setting an example of curiosity, creativity, and freedom.

BREAST-FEEDING

Creativity is at the heart of a family's well-being. Positive thoughts and words contribute to a healthy climate in the family, provided the father of the newborn participates in the creative venture of childbirth and raising the child, beginning with hugging and kissing both the mother and the child during feeding. The involvement of men in breast-feeding and teaching the baby its very first skills starts when he openly shows affection and kindness toward the baby's mother, his beloved. The family bond is further strengthened if the mother and father sit opposite each other holding the baby in their arms (or opposite the baby in a crib), as well as lying in each other's embrace during breast-feeding sessions. If the child is unwell or is teething, the Inner Smile meditation found in chapter 2 is recommended, as it sends virtuous emotions along with the appropriate color to the child; singing or playing an instrument enhances the virtue of this practice.

In *The Scientification of Love*, Michel Odent says,

> The taste of breast milk is always unique. In the first days after birth, it is not the same as in the following days. At the beginning of feeding, the milk does not taste like [it does] in the end. Morning milk is different from evening milk. The taste of milk depends on what the mother ate. Milk mixture, on the contrary, is always the same, from the first drop to the last, at any time of the day or night. Of course, the sense of taste begins to develop long before birth, because the taste of amniotic fluid that the baby swallows in the womb depends on what mother eats.

The spiritual and emotional qualities of breast milk depend on many factors: the woman's emotions, the security (or lack of) she feels in her environment, and the warmth and mutual understanding of her

140 Family Care

man. Colostrum and milk are hormonal because they are the result of infusions of hormones produced by a woman's endocrine glands. If a breast-feeding woman gets pleasure from the process, it causes her to produce extra endorphins, the hormones of satisfaction and happiness. This energy is attractive to her loving partner, whose attendance at the time of breast-feeding increases the libido of both partners. Heartfelt empathy, compassion, and love are absorbed by the baby along with the milk of the baby's mother. All these qualities are amplified by the loving attention of the father. The act of breast-feeding is inseparable from conception, pregnancy, and birth. It is through this cultivation of the virtues of the organs through breast-feeding that the body and spirit is instilled with health and chi, and the family's identity is born. If these processes are allowed to go on undisturbed by social expectations and taboos, then the woman rejuvenates her own health and that of her family. The baby's stem cells are stimulated by the positive vibrations of the mother and the father, insuring happiness, health, and longevity. This is confirmed by Taoist practices, which return a person to a state of physical, mental, and emotional balance.

Marina's Field Notes

The Inner Smile meditation helped me get back in touch with my two-year-old son when I had to interrupt his nursing. We were living in Vermont at the time. It was a cold winter, and the children spent a lot of time either by the fireplace (which wasn't always easy to get going) in our rented summer house or in the city library, in a warm playroom. Unexpectedly I was summoned to a seminar in Moscow, and at that time I was still actively breast-feeding my youngest son (it is not preferable to wean babies during winter). When I returned, my son met me with bitter crying and pushed me away because I had betrayed our closeness for such a long time, as the trip ended up lasting six weeks. After a few minutes I managed to hug him and I began to smile at him with my heart, and then he finally smiled, unbuttoned my blouse, and took to my breast. I began to hum the healing sounds, and the milk flowed like a river. We were reunited. I breast-fed him until he was four and a half years old, and having learned this valuable lesson from my young son, I thereafter always took him on all of my trips. Only once I went to India without him for a short while. But we had the internet at that time, so before going to bed we would do the healing sounds together.

The Subtle Energies of Mother's Milk

Again and again we return to the bubbling source of life—the breast. Female breasts are a source of eroticism, given to a woman for breast-feeding and to enhance her beauty; they can attract a man and help him open his heart. What could be more beautiful than breast-feeding the fruit of one's love in the embrace of the baby's father!

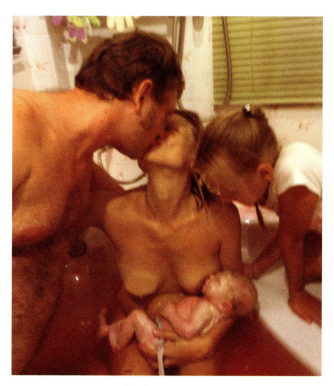

Fig. 6.3. Breast-feeding within the family matrix

142 Family Care

But breasts also nourish subtle energy. A breast-feeding woman should understand that the intimate relationship with her child allows for the strongest connection to the vibrations of the cosmos, as her pituitary, hypothalamus, and cerebellum receive the greatest amount of violet light, life-force energy, and cell reproduction stimulants. Gazing at the stars in the night sky during breast-feeding, without being distracted by phone calls or technology, is especially powerful for increasing the chi in breast milk.

At the time of feeding the child receives not only the most nutrient-dense form of life-giving energy, but also the necessary subconscious information about the essence of his incarnation. This occurs when the baby's eyes are in his mother's eyes and his heart has merged with his mother's heart. A mother rooted in her motherhood is connected to Mother Earth, who nourishes mother and child and all life forms. A woman who works the soil and plants grains and flower seeds, berries and herbs, is filled with the energy of the earth, which is very important during pregnancy and breast-feeding. Osho speaks of breast-feeding as a tantric privilege, an invitation to be in love with life. He believes that it is through a mother's milk that a child connects once again with Source, a connection that replaces the earlier connection through the umbilical cord. So the energy the child had previously received through his navel now flows through his mouth. Osho believed that if a child does not get nourishment from his mother's milk, his vital energy will remain weak later in life. It is true that babies can in fact be fed in other ways, but it is that connection with the mother's heart as she holds a child to her breast that promises a long and happy life. Those children who never drank their mother's milk will likely not be able to achieve great bliss in life, as it is through the mother's milk that the child discovers the taste of life. This maternal dew activates vital enzymes that assist in the assimilation of physical as well as pranic (energetic) food. If the mother softly sings a lullaby to her child while nursing, the child's nervous system calms, which helps the vital juices to flow through vital channels.

Children are very receptive to their mother's touch during breast-feeding. Tactile stimulation contributes to good digestion and balanced emotions. Our ability to absorb nutrition and eliminate what isn't needed is directly related to our feelings and emotions. Our cells are imprinted with all the vibrations that flow through mother's milk. Parental love and mutual understanding during lactation protect the baby from allergies and eczema, which could appear due to a mother rejecting breast-feeding or harboring negative emotions during feeding. That is the beauty of the Inner Smile meditation found in chapter 2, which allows the mother to pass the loving vibrations of the virtues to her baby eye to eye, as well as through her milk.

While breast-feeding it is possible to practice the Microcosmic Orbit, found in chapter 2. You visualize raising the energy of the earth up through the feet to the sex organs, and then flex the muscles, with the breath letting it pass along the spine to the top, connecting with the cosmic energy.

After practicing the Microcosmic Orbit, you can expand the energy to the entire cosmos by feeling the violet color of the constellation Ursa Major and connecting with the pole stars Thuban and Vega,

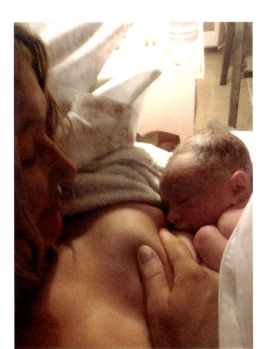

Fig. 6.4. Breast-feeding and connecting to the cosmos

144 *Family Care*

and distributing this cosmic energy to the glands and organs of both yourself and your baby. In this way you can connect your own energy and that of your baby with the planetary mind and like-minded people, using this energy for healing the planet and ourselves.

Weaning

It may seem counterintuitive, but when a child first begins to teethe at anywhere from six months to a year, breast-feeding is especially necessary for the child's comfort. Often mothers refuse at this point because the child starts to playfully bite on the nipples. However, the eyes and thoughts of the mother can prevent or soften this moment. Scolding the child should be avoided; it is better to correct with a small bite to the plump palm of the baby's hand, where there are certain receptors of understanding located that will help the child understand. Patient parents raise clever children.

Weaning is always very stressful for a baby. Its emotional life as well as its immune system and other physiological systems are established during the period of breast-feeding. If weaning occurs before the one-year mark, the reaction to introducing new foods can be unpredictable. New foods should be introduced along with partial breast-feeding, which allows the new enzymes to be better absorbed. It is also important for the family to bless the food before partaking. Ceremonies are important to us in all aspects of life. The ceremony of drinking mother's milk and eating one's first solid food is as important as the ritual of conception and birth. The nature of life shines in all these moments.

📝 Marina's Field Notes

Today we were welcomed by the fauna and flora of Santa Barbara, California. On the streets and at the pier, the laughter of children crystallized in spaces of love. Parents were holding their children's hands or carrying them on their shoulders or in slings or pushing them in strollers. Everyone greeted us and smiled back at our greetings. The energy of parenthood and childhood attracts nature: we couldn't help but notice all the birds in the sky, seals basking on a sandy beach, a giant sea lion trumpeting his greeting, and the splashing of gulls and pelicans at the water's edge. In the ocean we saw dolphins and whales. The children were so attracted to them, and they felt the children, too.

Not so long ago I met a family with three children and a pregnant mother. They turned to me, fearful of a fourth cesarean section. The parents were also concerned about the older kids' health issues. We started talking, and it turned out that the father of the family didn't want the mother to breast-feed for fear that she might lose her sexual appetite, and the woman was worried about the shape of her breasts. Why does this happen to families in culturally developed countries? Lack of information, infantilism, the desire to maintain comfort . . . And where does this kind of limited thinking come from? When did the wisdom of our ancestors and the knowledge that women have held for eons get replaced by the recommendations of the medical system?

A man who wasn't breast-fed or whose feeding was cut short may want to remain a child into adulthood (the so-called Peter Pan syndrome). One of the reasons for this is that the final formation of the brain occurred without the closing moment of weaning at the age of one year or later. This affects the physiology of digestion and a tendency to emotional conflict. For the boy who did not know closeness to his mother through breast-feeding, his attitude toward women in general and motherhood in particular will suffer. He may perceive breasts solely as erotic objects, without any connection to the heart, maybe even becoming obsessed with big "boobs." This affects relationships, as this man is searching for a connection with his heart energy through the energy of the breasts, which will ultimately lead to disappointment and the endless quest to find another, better, big-busted woman who can fulfill his frozen need for the early nurturing that breast-feeding would have provided.

Perhaps women who as babies were deprived of breast-feeding or whose feeding was cut short will tend to be critical of their breasts, unhappy with their size or shape. Such women may be more likely to reject breast-feeding their own children or might choose to enhance their breasts through surgery, which reduces sensitivity and impairs breast-feeding should they choose to do so. If the surgery is performed in the best possible way and the mammary glands are not damaged, the pain of feeding will nevertheless continue beyond the first few days, as breast implants compress and change the temperature of the mammary glands. Sometimes these women do not feed their babies for very long and do not bring harmony to the feeding process. It seems that for some women no arguments will stop them from keeping what they consider to be the focus of their sex appeal.

POTTY TRAINING

Taoist self-massage removes the stagnant energies of negative emotions and rejuvenates the vital organs to create a positive emotional state. For newborns, this rejuvenating massage is naturally activated in the eagle position, where the parents hold the baby in a squatting position over a potty or a basin, bending its legs at the knees and supporting the baby's feet with the palms of their hands. This also happens to be the best position for potty-training.

Where people live in simple, natural environments and rural settings—which tend to be places where the intuitive way of life is cultivated and traditional values are honored—the mother is always the child's first model. In traditional cultures, women working in the field or in the jungle with their babies tied on their backs would intuitively know when to set the baby down for a potty break as guided by their own needs, and the child would quickly get used to synchronizing with the mother. The child effortlessly learned to hold urine by contracting the muscles, and then learned to release in the eagle position, thereby training the muscles that will later be used in a future of sexual creativity.

Family Care 147

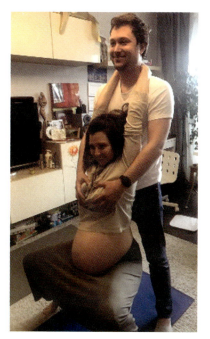 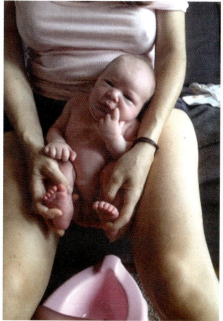

Fig. 6.5. Parents and infant in eagle pose or squatting position, similar to the position for emptying the bladder or bowels.

If this process takes place in a natural position and with the support of the mother, her voice mimicking the sound of running water, then the baby gets pleasure from a bowel movement and emptying the bladder.

Positive emotions should be present in all endeavors appropriate to the age and needs of a developing brain and the nervous and musculoskeletal systems. If, for example, the baby is scolded by his mother or father or grandmother or teacher for wetting his pants, the child is shamed, and this is when the child begins to repress. If the child has been successful on the potty and is praised for it, then he can bask in a sense of pride in this accomplishment; he is open to new conquests in this world full of wonders, without feeling fear, guilt, or shame. And the world really is full of wonders and joy, mother's kisses and her smile, and the big, strong arms of his father playfully tossing him high in the sky.

THE VALUE OF PLAY

It is important that parents inspire children at every stage of their development. This is where play can be so effective. Parents should themselves play, continuing their love games with each other and allowing the children to experience the joy of their play as well as their own fun in playing. There are musical potty chairs and singing toys; handmade wooden or cloth toys such as cars and dolls; all sorts of interesting toys with rings, ladders, and bars; and realistic-looking houses with various moving parts.

Children up to a certain age often experience flying in their dreams. This means that they have not yet separated from their life before birth, and free-floating in space is still within the realm of possibility. Such flying is inherent to our subtle bodies. As life gets progressively more mundane and materially oriented, which comes with age, we are less likely to fly; we also feel inexplicable happiness less and less. Taoist practices allow us to once again experience the joy of flying like we did when we were kids. Of course, these practices need to be learned and practiced regularly as part of our everyday life.

 ## Astral Vertical Flight Training

Play is not just for kids—parents can play too. If it has been a long time since you experienced the joy of flying in your dreams (or in your meditations), try the following exercise from the Universal Healing Tao.

1. Start at the point above the top of your head, the location of your higher spiritual body.
2. Rotate your perception in a circle, from the area between the eyebrows (the third eye), and rotate above your head parallel to the ground.
3. Acceleration will create the sense of flying in space.

4. Practice this once a week when you feel calm and carefree. The best time is 15 to 20 minutes after other meditations. If practiced at night, the activity will continue during sleep. In this flying exercise it is preferable to keep the physical body in an upright position (until sleep).

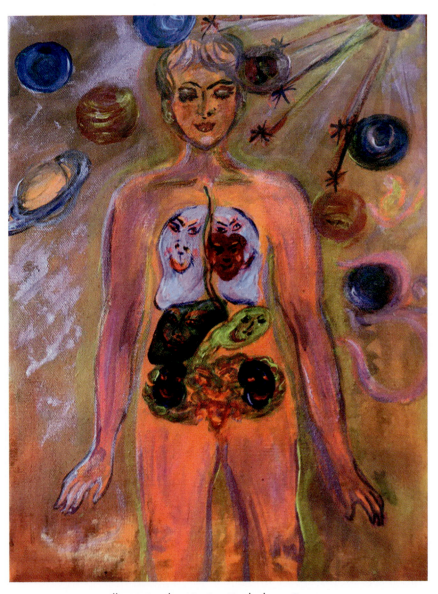

Illustration by Marina Dadasheva-Drown

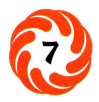

The Coming of the Indigo Children

Indigo is a deep blue with a hint of violet. It is the color that is connected to the third eye chakra, a potent spiritual center that is all about intuition, clairvoyance, clairaudience, and clairsentience. It relates to meditation and our higher selves. So we can say that indigo represents the knowledge of the soul and connecting to the Divine. This is a hallmark of the Indigo Children.

A child is very sensitive by nature and is constantly under the influence of its environment and the many moods created by the relationship between the parents. That's why the modern taboo against a child experiencing the loving feelings between parents does not contribute to a very healthy family matrix: children need to see evidence of love and intimacy—they need to see their parents hugging and kissing, and see them exchange kind words and kind actions. If the family matrix is basically one of conflict, it will result in grief and the destruction of love for the whole family. Children from such dysfunctional families grow up to be skeptical about marriage and procreation. In extreme cases such a person might be cruel to animals or think that good doesn't exist. Or in the absence of a loving parental role model they might try to prove their worth by accumulating material wealth.

This is why all cultures and religions nurture strong families and stable marriages. The key to a healthy family is that all members respect one another. As Karl Marx, a German intellectual and Communist philosopher said, "The culture of civilized society is determined by the relationship between men and women, and especially by the respect that men have for women." Marx grew up in a large family, as have many notable scientists, educators, and esoteric philosophers who have changed the world. They came from families that preserved the tradition of passing down knowledge and skills to their children, where the father and mother were respected and loved by their many children. Support and solidarity are what determine the quality of family wealth.

Joseph Chilton Pearce, in *The Biology of Transcendence*, talks about how the mother in particular "creates and brings the child into the world [and] also models for him, educates him, and leads him forth into knowledge. She, then, must be one with the knowledge of that greatest and most priceless good news of who we are: one with our creator."[1] This is a two-way street, as the mother and the child each have something to contribute to the other. The child as a newly incarnated soul has a more recent connection with Source, which benefits the mother; for the mother it is her love and her commitment to developing her own higher faculties that benefit the child. Pearce says,

> Just as creator and created give rise to each other, so do parent and child. The intriguing thing about this dynamic is that the child awakens in the parent ancient vistas of knowledge vital to the ongoing dynamic, in order that she [the mother] might awaken the same in that child. Mirror to mirror again. So a truly new beginning must begin not with the child, but with the future mother, so that she may be awakened to the awareness of who she is, that she is in charge of her life, preferably before she conceives and critically before she gives birth.[2]

This is what nurtures the arrival of the Indigo Children, who are highly creative and can see through the established norms of society. They are old souls who have been called in at this pivotal time in human history to shake up the modern world and pave the way for future generations to create peace and harmony for all.

The Chi Kung Melting Embrace is the quintessence of the Healing Tao and a guide to conscious parenting, which is a precondition for the incarnation of a conscious being such as an Indigo. This meditation promotes good feelings, resolves any conflicts, and creates trust. It also creates space to call in a new soul if the couple wishes to conceive, and if there are already children, it cultivates a good atmosphere in the family, where children, their parents, and other elders are respected and taken care of.

A good family atmosphere happens when parents encourage creativity in their children; this makes family life a symphony. The notes of healthy sexuality based on trust, common aspirations, fulfilling work, and sufficient leisure are very important in the symphony. All of this is based in love. By creating love, we create a space for children where

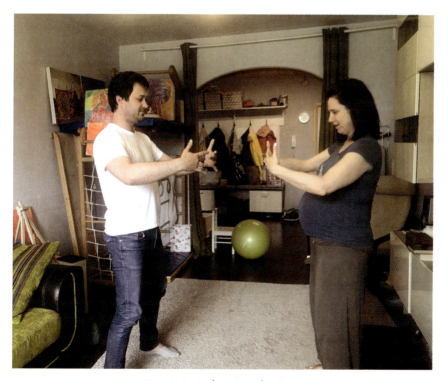

Fig. 7.1. Embracing the Tree

there is no fear, no resentment, no distrust, and where their higher faculties can emerge naturally.

Chi Kung Melting Embrace

The Melting Embrace creates a stream of love in the Microcosmic Orbit, in which the exchange of breaths between partners synchronizes their orbits and creates a protective cocoon of love for both the couple and the in-utero child. This meditation can also be done if your intention is to conceive, and you wish to create a loving space in which to do so.

1. The man and woman stand in front of each other about one foot apart with feet parallel, shoulder-width apart, in the pose called Embracing the Tree (See fig 7.1). If one of the partners is taller, he or she should slightly bend the knees so that the partners are facing each other.
2. Both partners step toward each other until they are just a few inches apart.
3. Each partner lowers the right hand to the level of the tailbone of the other partner, while the left hand covers their partner's Jade Pillow, the area at the base of the skull. This position is heart to heart, belly to belly (or tan tien to tan tien), pubis to pubis, and lips to ear, so you can whisper words of love to each other.
4. Begin to synchronize your breathing using the Abdominal Breathing exercise (see chapter 1). One partner inhales while the other exhales, so as one partner expands the belly on an inhalation, the other partner pulls the belly in toward the spine on an exhalation. The technique is very interesting for pregnant couples, as it simulates the baby penetrating into the belly of the father.
5. Visualize an egg of love being created between the partners that the baby bathes in. This protective energy remains with the baby after birth. It is especially important for the partners to maintain this ritual of love contact until their child attains puberty.

The Coming of the Indigo Children 155

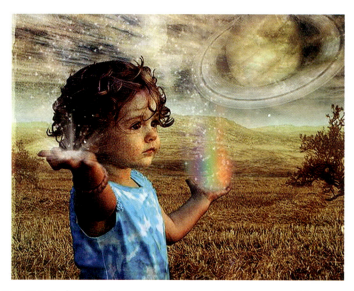

Fig. 7.2. Indigo Children are an upgraded prototype of humanity. Their aura appears as a royal blue. They are on a mission to shift humanity.

HERALDING THE ARRIVAL OF THE INDIGOS

In our times, the legacy of the famous Orientalist, Theosophist, and artist Nicholas Roerich (1874–1947) has gained worldwide recognition. Roerich and his remarkable wife, Helena, a co-partner in their work together, transmitted the philosophy of Agni Yoga, or "Mergence with Divine Fire." Designed as a daily practice, Agni Yoga, a yoga of fiery energy, teaches that the evolution of planetary consciousness is an attainable aspiration for humankind. This was many years before the appearance of the first Indigo Children in the 1970s. The Roerichs considered Agni Yoga to be the synthesis of all yogas. They were models of the philosophy they espoused. Nicholas Roerich called his wife *Drugina*, Russian for "friend." Helena Roerich was a loving assistant in their work together as the heralds of humane ethics. In Roerich's work, we find the first mention of extraordinary children being born from the ocean, their skin glowing with a violet hue.

156 The Coming of the Indigo Children

The artistic and philosophical heritage of Nikolas and Helena Roerich and their sons, Svetoslav and Yuri, is full of hope for the birth of the new humanity, supported by the mahatmas of Shambhala and the future buddha, Maitreya, with the Mother of the World asserting a feminine humanism and with Helena Roerich as the prototype.

The Roerichs' legacy set the stage for the appearance of the Indigo Children, although it wasn't until much later that the phenomenon was described almost simultaneously by two scientists who in their individual work paved the way for this knowledge to come forth in the present time: Drunvalo Melchizedek, the author of *The Ancient Secret of the Flower of Life*; and Lee Carroll, who channels the entity known as Kryon and who wrote *The Indigo Children: The New Kids Have Arrived*.

Melchizedek describes in detail the phenomenon of children who see and feel differently from anyone else, who first appeared in China, then in Russia, and later in Europe and America. He describes the way these extraordinary children look at the world and puts forward the concept of the thinking and feeling heart that can see the future and transmit healing impulses to other people.

In ancient times in China, this kind of knowledge was cultivated and used to strengthen the power of the empire in its invincibility. This was reflected in the development of the Healing Tao, with its ability to open energy channels to store and conserve energy. Throughout the stages of conception and conscious pregnancy and by using Taoist practices, women then gave birth to children not only without experiencing pain but in orgasmic ecstasy. Knowing the notes of Taoist Healing Love largely contributed to this. When the ancient peoples of the East lost this sacred knowledge there came the onset of brutal wars, in which priority was given to men in bodily combat, while the previous practices of women that trained them in the use of their sacred muscles and the indestructible spiritual potential of the heart were quashed. This is when women lost their knowledge of the natural regulation of fertility through Taoist practices and began to give birth in pain.

Spiritual masters in Tibet and India, however, managed to preserve the secret knowledge of the chakras, the spinal channels (the Ida, Pingala, and Sushumna), the flow of kundalini energy, and the life force known as *prana* or *chi*. These teachings on the flow of energy and the powers of sexuality have only resurfaced in the West in relatively recent times, which is fitting given the perilous times in which we are living and the need for higher consciousness to develop in humanity. These powers have a transformative effect. They can be used to conceive wonderful children in love ecstasy or can be transformed to gain spiritual knowledge and physical well-being, and can be parlayed into any number of creative endeavors. Thanks to what was previously hidden knowledge, which has been revealed to us through the Universal Healing Tao, a pregnant couple can instill the codes of perfect health and superpower abilities at the chromosomal level of the future human they are co-creating.

It is very important that parents who practice the Universal Healing Tao do not stop practicing once the child has been born. Continuing the practices secures the capabilities of the newborn, who live directly in the parents' field up until the age of puberty. It is thus very important to breast-feed your baby, and by so providing the mother's elixir of love, awakening in the child the subconscious knowledge of the true values of life.

In Tibetan and Vedic cultures it was believed that the in-utero child has not seven but twelve chakras, which connect directly to the twelve centers of the Earth and its kundalini, much like the umbilical cord that feeds the baby with the energy of the placenta. With these spiritual centers we can assume that clairvoyance is possible in all stages of life, from the zygote to the baby. In many traditional cultures it is believed that shamans retain visions from the period of their infancy thanks to their cultural milieu, which fosters extrasensory capabilities as part of healing.

We often meet children who have not blocked their superpowers, but rather have developed them thanks to encouragement from their aware parents or teachers. It is not easy for parents and

158 The Coming of the Indigo Children

mentors to be brought up by such children, which is exactly what happens—adults become their disciples! This is the role that our own children can play in our lives if we allow them to. Most schools, even the better ones, do not foster natural intelligence. Starting at around three years of age, considered to be the time when gender is established, it is preferable to raise a child in the loving embrace of the family, avoiding things like guilt and shame, which pediatricians say dull the child's virtuous qualities of kindness, empathy, and compassion. Joseph Chilton Pearce devoted his books *Magical Child*, *Magical Child Matures*, and *The Biology of Transcendence* to this topic, approaching it from both a scientific and an esoteric angle. He brings our attention to the fact that intellectual development in children is inhibited when prohibitions and coercion are used. This is becoming more pronounced now with mandated vaccinations and the rise in cesarean section births.

THE MISSION OF THE INDIGOS

The philosophy and meditations of the Universal Healing Tao assert that our life is a microcosm subject to the laws of the cosmos. Humans are connected to the planets and stars. The ancient treatises of the Tao that came into existence even before the time of the Yellow Emperor (ca. 2700 BCE) talk about the strong influence that the Ursa Major constellation and all the celestial bodies closest to it have on us. This includes the Pole Stars, Thuban, and Vega, as well as Mercury, the planet that directly creates the energy of our kidneys and their companions, the sex organs. The vibrations of the colors that emanate from those stars reflect on the back of the skull, and from there they are sent to the crown of the head, impacting the pituitary gland, the pineal gland, the cerebellum, the hypothalamus, and the rest of the glands—the thyroid, parathyroid, thymus, pancreas, adrenal glands, and sex organs. Further effects on the other organs occur through the innumerable sound and color waves that fill our lives to create positive emotions within us that are returned to the cosmos.

The Coming of the Indigo Children 159

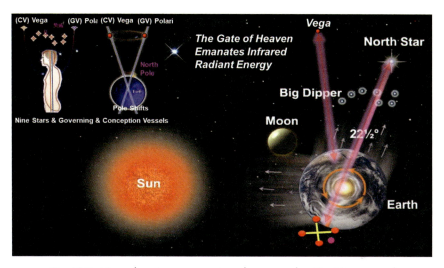

Fig. 7.3. Map showing connections between the Big Dipper and the North Star with the glands of the human brain

Thanks to the balance of positively and negatively charged particles in the universe, new galactic life is created in this way. The same thing happens in the microcosm of the human body when we procreate. Yin and yang lead a man and a woman to sexual arousal and the desire to create a love fusion, where the energy has enough power to make conception happen.

Let's return to the Indigo Child, the subject of Lee Carroll's first book in the Kryon series, *The Indigo Children*. In this wonderful book, Carroll says,

> The desires of an Indigo are very simple: more love and favorable conditions for the development, reasonable mentoring, and freedom to express their bright individuality. In return, our world will receive gifts that are hard to dream of:
>
> > World arm in arm together the world and I
> > And all the people black and white, and all whales
> > Waltzing in the sea, all dolphins
> > Gliding in the surf

160 The Coming of the Indigo Children

Hand in hand go together, and guess what?
Why war?
Why the anger?
Why the hate?
The world and I and all creatures of the Earth together
forever hand in hand.

A poem of an Indigo girl, Sarah Berkeley, at age ten[3]

THE TEACHINGS OF THE DOLPHINS

Water, when combined with positive affirmations, can change the structure of even our own memory. This is exactly why we need water births. Kids raised by mindful parents make our entire generation whole and take us away from the illusions of the medical system. Let's raise our consciousness and not impose our unrealized aspirations and traumas on our children. For adults who experienced a traumatic birth or a traumatic early childhood, rebirthing, especially when done in water, dissolves any resistance you might have to experiencing your innate strength and pre-birth purity of being. This increases planetary compassion and helps us prepare for a future populated by Indigo Children.

Let's consider dolphins, whose energies are connected to the new generation of children born in water, be it at home or in the ocean. When we hear dolphin songs, we feel something unusually and even painfully touching and mixed with the mysticism of oceanic sunrises and sunsets, something that touches our deepest heart vibrations. We're overcome with a prayerful feeling of ecstasy. Mantra, Yantra, and Tantra are in this same category of invocatory singing of love and compassion. A unique feature of dolphins is their absolute love for all things. They are incapable of resentment, hostility, revenge, and desperation. Instead, we see the love and power of their flights, their fast and smooth movements, the way they greet the sun and people, and the humane way they eat, with gratitude. There are tales among the peoples living near the coast, legends about these amazing, loving beauties who save people from drowning and help women get pregnant and give birth to children in orgasmic ecstasy.

Many pregnant women in their dreams and meditations see these incredibly peaceful teachers of humanity with their unborn babies. There is also a belief that every water-born baby has as its leader a dolphin.

📝 Marina's Field Notes

During my pregnancies I swam with bottlenose dolphins in the Black Sea, and in my dreams I saw big, white, graceful dolphins and smaller pink dolphins. Later, on one of the islands in the Surat Thani area in southern Thailand, I met a rose-colored, glowing fish-bird that was hovering over the water in an acrobatic flip. And in the Mexican water depths as well as near Santa Barbara there are beluga whales. There are a lot of beautiful children in these areas. A lot of them are in the water, surfing and sailing and paddling canoes. Sea, sandy beaches, mountains in sunbeams at the dawn, a rainbow over the breakwaters, sea lions and seals lounging by the water, pelicans and gulls diving for the fish in the water . . . And children—smiling and laughing children of different ages and colors, and their calm, independent parents . . .

That's how dolphins see the world, sending us their love songs despite the human folly of Japanese dolphin hunters, captivity in aquatic zoos, and the military use of dolphins as rocket-launch vehicles. Dolphins continue to teach us with their love because that is their purpose. Since the brain of a dolphin is not subject to gravity and their water environment supports the extrasensory capabilities of its frontal lobes, which contribute to transcendental states, dolphins are absolute pacifists.

A female dolphin gives birth in the depths of the ocean, in the intimacy of a dance with her partner. The whole pack waits and sings. When the baby bursts out of the mother's womb, spinning in circles, an adult female or the mother herself pushes the baby to the surface.

The baby's first breath, the mother's colostrum, the soft delivery of the placenta, the maternal meal, and the completion with a ritual song—it's no secret that dolphins are very sexual, just like we humans. The vibrations created by a female dolphin in labor are orgasmic. Like in humans, the entrance to her secret gate does not close during pregnancy, so the dolphin couple saturates the world's oceans with their love, attracting the attention of the world with their mesmerizing mating songs. Live in a field of dolphins, visualize their love dances, witness the birth of dolphin pups, and your life will become much more beautiful.

CREATING LOVE WITH LOVE

"To be or not to be?" Nowadays this rhetorical question of Shakespeare's Hamlet is as relevant as ever, not so much on the individual level, but on the planetary level. Will our planet Earth survive? Will its human population survive, or will the soulless reptilian brain take charge once again? The mindset of "Why even give birth to children when the end is near," referring to the destruction of the environment, inhumanity, diseases, and overpopulation, are the reasons that are given to justify callousness, sex instead of love, and birth control pills that change the DNA. This line of thinking that goes "Why breed if we're all going to die?" is very close to "Why live if we're all going to die?" There are a lot of contradictions in this dystopian viewpoint! This person does not just want to simply survive, he wants to live in prosperity and fame, to live better than others and have fun at all costs, even if it entails violence, oppression, murder, and destruction of the planet's natural resources. Of course if there were no people who hold a different, more truthful and positive worldview, we would have long ago disappeared from the face of the Earth, having turned into lava or cosmic dust.

So what saves humanity from its inhumane activities? The forces of nature, the animal world, higher intelligence, and the arrival of children of the new dimension, the Indigos. If we stop giving birth to children naturally, don't raise them humanely, and don't allow them to come into contact with the higher civilization of the dolphins, we are unlikely to remain people who are capable of feeling love and compassion. And so, despite all the currently fashionable ideas around celibacy, and intentional childlessness, a woman ends up feeling happy at the idea of standing beside her man, her perfect consort, dreaming of their future child . . .

Whatever we are like in our marriage partnership today, tomorrow this will exist in our child. If we are aggressive, our child will be aggressive; if we are angry, our child will be angry. If we are weak and spineless, if we see ourselves as victims, our child will also be a victim. To prevent this from happening we must learn kindness and acceptance of different points of view and different ways of living. This is what marriage as well as parenthood is all about. None of us is born a wife or a husband; we find the opportunity to become one, to invite another person into our life and respect their right to be who they are, to be different from us, and different in love, sorrow, and joy. Unselfish respect and acceptance in love can only be taught by children, which is why they come in due time, as assistants, teachers, and disciples.

Joseph Chilton Pearce maintains that we have five different neural structures or "brains" within us, three of them in our head. The three neural structures in our head chart the evolution of consciousness in human beings: the old reptilian brain, the mammalian brain, and the human brain. Each time we move forward in our evolution we do so to overcome the shortcomings of the previous stage of development. "Each neural creation opened life to vast new realms of possibility and, at the same time, brought new problems, thus calling once again for 'rising and going beyond' through the creation of yet another neural structure," he says. "Thus, while we refer to transcendence in rather mystical, ethereal terms to the intelligence of life, transcendence may be simply the next intelligent move to make."[4]

The latest research from the HeartMath Institute confirms that our fifth brain (the fourth is in the gut) is found in our heart. In using this fifth brain and "thinking with the heart," we profoundly affect the nature of our conscious awareness, and in so doing we shape our collective reality. This is fully supported by the revelations of quantum physics and is the key to humanity's transcendence. And it has always been so. Love is the heart's intelligence, and when we create new life with it, we create ever more love, compassion, joy, fun, exhilaration, and peace within us and in the world.

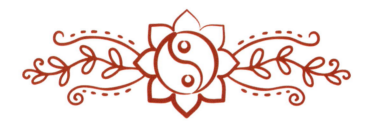

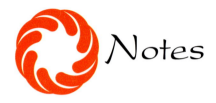

Notes

Chapter 2. Knowing Your Own Sexuality
1. Tower, "Stress and stem cells."

Chapter 3. The Alchemy of Conception
1. Roerich, *Brotherhood*, 113.

Chapter 4. Pregnancy
1. Thomas Verny, in Lipton, *Biology of Belief*.
2. Grof, *Realms of Human Unconscious*.
3. Pearce, *Biology of Transcendence*, 134.

Chapter 5. Birth
1. Matsumoto and Shirahashi, "Novel perspectives."
2. Moyer, "Power of Placenta."
3. Damianos, Xu, Kalin, and Kalinichenko, "Placental tissue stem cells."
4. McBride, "Legacy of Distorted Love."

Chapter 6. Family Care
1. Baron, "Michel Odent: 'How long can humanity survive now?'"

Chapter 7. The Coming of the Indigo Children
1. Pearce, *Biology of Transcendence*, 247.
2. Pearce, *Biology of Transcendence*, 248.
3. Carroll, *Indigo Children*.
4. Pearce, *Biology of Transcendence*, 4.

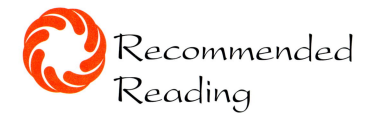

Recommended Reading

OTHER RELATED BOOKS BY MANTAK CHIA

Awaken Healing Energy through the Tao: The Taoist Secret of Circulating Internal Power. Aurora Press, 1999.
Bone Marrow Nei Kung: Taoist Techniques for Rejuvenating the Blood and Bone. Rochester, VT: Destiny Books, 2006.
Cosmic Healing I: Cosmic Chi Kung. Universal Healing Tao Publications, 2001.
Fusion of the Five Elements: Meditations for Transforming Negative Emotions. Rochester, VT: Destiny Books 2007.
Healing Light of the Tao: Foundational Practices to Awaken Chi Energy. Rochester, VT: Destiny Books, 2008.
Healing Love through the Tao: Cultivating Female Sexual Energy. Rochester, VT: Destiny Books, 2005.
Iron Shirt Chi Kung. Rochester, VT: Destiny Books, 2006.
Karsai Nei Tsang: Therapeutic Massage for the Sexual Organs. Rochester, VT: Destiny Books, 2011.
The Six Healing Sounds Taoist Techniques for Balancing Chi. Rochester, VT: Destiny Books, 2009.
———, and Anna Margolina. *Chi Kung for Radiant Skin: Taoist Secrets for Inner and Outer Beauty.* Rochester, VT: Destiny Books, 2022.
———, and William U. Wei. *Cosmic Nutrition: The Taoist Approach to Health and Longevity.* Rochester, VT: Destiny Books, 2012.
———, and Aisha Sieburth. *Life Pulse Massage: Taoist Techniques for Enhanced Circulation and Detoxification.* Rochester, VT: Destiny Books, 2015.

168 Recommended Readings

———, and Kris Deva North. *Taoist Shaman Practices from the Wheel of Life.* Rochester, VT: Destiny Books, 2011.

———, and Christine Harkness-Giles. *Taoist Secrets of Eating for Balance: Your Personal Program for Five-Element Nutrition.* Rochester, VT: Destiny Books, 2019.

———, and Michael Winn. *Taoist Secrets of Love: Cultivating Male Sexual Energy.* Aurora Press, 2016.

INFORMATION ABOUT HEALTH AND SEXUALITY

Baron, Saskia. "Michel Odent: 'How long can humanity survive now?'" *Guardian,* Oct. 7, 2017.

Carroll, Lee. *The Indigo Children: The New Kids Have Arrived.* Carlsbad, CA: Hay House, 1999.

Damianos, Andreas, Kui Xu, Gregory T. Kalin, and Vladimir V. Kalinichenko. "Placental tissue stem cells and their role in neonatal diseases." *Seminars in Fetal and Neonatal Medicine* 27, no. 1 (2022).

Draelos, Zoe, and Peter T. Pugliese. *Physiology of the Skin,* 3rd ed. Carol Stream, IL: Allured Publishing Corporation, 2011.

Grof, Stanislav. *Realms of Human Unconscious: Observations from LSD Research.* New York: E. P. Dutton, 1976.

Hawkins, David R. *Power Vs. Force: The Hidden Determinants of Human Behavior.* Carlsbad, CA: Hay House, 2002.

Lipton, Bruce. *The Biology of Belief: Unleashing the Power of Consciousness, Matter, and Miracles.* Carlsbad, CA: Hay House, 2008.

Margolina, Anna, and Elena Hernandez. *New Cosmetology: The Foundational Principles of Modern Cosmetology* [In Russian]. Moscow: Cosmetics and Medicine Publishing, 2012.

———. *New Cosmetology: The Foundational Principles of Modern Cosmetology* [In Russian]. Moscow: Cosmetics and Medicine Publishing, 2015.

———, and Anna Petrukhina. *Lipid Barrier and Cosmetics* [in Russian]. Moscow: Cosmetics and Medicine Publishing, 2003.

Matsumoto, Shin-Ichiro, and Kiyohiko Shirahashi. "Novel perspectives on the influence of the lunar cycle on the timing of full-term human births." *Chronobiology International* 37, no. 7 (2020): 1082–89.

McBride, Karyl. "The Legacy of Distorted Love: Post-Romantic Stress." *Psychology Today*, Feb. 10, 2012.

Melchizedek, Drunvalo. *Living in the Heart: How to Enter into the Sacred Space within the Heart*. Light Technology Publishing, 2003.

Meneghetti, Antonio. *Pedagogia ontopsicologica*. Ontopsicologia Editrice, 2007.

Moyer, Hollie S. "The Power of Placenta for Hemorrhage Control." *Midwifery Today* 112 (2015).

Odent, Michel. *The Scientification of Love*. Free Association Books, 1999.

———. *Water and Sexuality*. 2014

Pandey, Rajbali. *Hindu Samskaras: Socio-Religious Study of the Hindu Sacraments*. India: Motilal Banarsidass Publishers, 2013.

Pearce, Joseph Chilton. *The Biology of Transcendence: A Blueprint of the Human Experience*. Rochester, VT: Park Street Press, 2004.

Pickart, Loren, Anna Margolina, and Idelle Musiek. *Reverse Skin Aging: What Copper Peptides Can Do for You*. Cape San Juan Press/Summit Associates International, 2015.

Roerich, Nikolas. *Brotherhood 1937*. Whitefish, MT: Kessinger Reprints, 2006.

Schueller, Randy, and Perry Romanowski. *Beginning Cosmetic Chemistry: Practical Knowledge for the Cosmetic Industry*. Carol Stream, IL: Allured Publishing Corporation, 2009.

Tower, John. "Stress and stem cells." *Wiley Interdisciplinary Reviews Developmental Biology* 1, no. 6 (2012): 789–802.

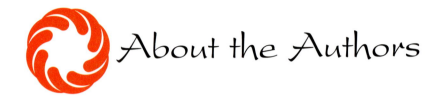

About the Authors

MANTAK CHIA

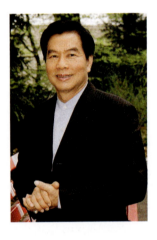

Mantak Chia has been studying the Taoist approach to life since childhood. His mastery of this ancient knowledge, enhanced by his study of other disciplines, has resulted in the development of the Universal Healing Tao system, which is now taught throughout the world.

Mantak Chia was born in Thailand to Chinese parents in 1944. When he was six years old, he learned from Buddhist monks how to sit and "still the mind." While in grammar school he learned traditional Thai boxing, and he soon went on to acquire considerable skill in aikido, yoga, and Tai Chi. His studies of the Taoist way of life began in earnest when he was a student in Hong Kong, ultimately leading to his mastery of a wide variety of esoteric disciplines, thanks to the guidance of several masters, including Master Yi Eng (I Yun), Master Meugi, Master Cheng Yao-Lun, and Master Pan Yu. To better understand the mechanisms behind healing energy, he also studied Western anatomy and medical sciences.

Master Chia has taught his system of healing and energizing practices to tens of thousands of students and trained more than three thousand instructors and practitioners throughout the world. Stemming from his teaching corps, there are established centers for Taoist study and training in many countries around the globe. Master Mantak Chia has been the only person named twice by the International Congress of Chinese Medicine and Qi Gong (Chi Kung) as Qi Gong Master of the Year (in 1990 and 2012). He was also listed as number 18 of the 100 most spiritually influential people in *The Watkins Review* in 2012.

MARINA DADASHEVA-DROWN

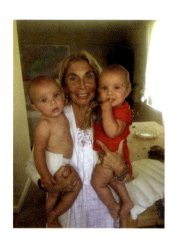

Marina Dadasheva-Drown, born in 1951, is a mother, wife, grandmother, and great-grandmother whose children were conceived and born free in love. She has devoted her life to healing people from birth injuries. She was born and grew up in Azerbaijan (where her first son was born) and graduated from Baku Slavic University. She worked as a teacher, journalist, and family psychologist in Moscow, Russia.

It was the birth of her own children that became the reason for her taking up the study of Tantra and Taoist and Vedic cultures, and she soon became well-known as a spiritual midwife. Having studied and mastered the medicine of traditional cultures, she became a student and colleague of Igor Charkovsky, a pioneer in home, water, and oceanic birth, with whom she also trained in children's yoga starting in 1990. She specializes in working with traumatized children and their parents using various types of breathing techniques, and she applies these practices in situations where there is problematic conception and childbirth.

In 1994 she met Master Mantak Chia and in that same year got married to his esteemed student Colin Campbell-Drown. Since 1996, with the birth of her tenth child, she began training and teaching the Healing Love Tao at Tao Garden in Thailand. In 2002, just as worldwide recognition of the methods of Healing Love Tao were blossoming in Europe, Asia, and the United States, she gave birth to her eleventh child.

172 About the Authors

Marina and her husband, Colin, the editor of many Mantak Chia books, continue their journey in the Universal Healing Tao, living and working in Thailand, at Master Chia's center there, as well as traveling throughout the world to teach Taoist methods of improving the health and longevity of people everywhere.

The Universal Healing Tao System and Training Center

THE UNIVERSAL HEALING TAO SYSTEM

The ultimate goal of Taoist practice is to transcend physical boundaries through the development of the soul and the spirit within the human being. That is also the guiding principle behind the Universal Healing Tao, a practical system of self-development that enables individuals to complete the harmonious evolution of their physical, mental, and spiritual bodies. Through a series of ancient Chinese meditative and internal energy exercises, the practitioner learns to increase physical energy, release tension, improve health, practice self-defense, and gain the ability to heal him- or herself and others. In the process of creating a solid foundation of health and well-being in the physical body, the practitioner also creates the basis for developing his or her spiritual potential by learning to tap into the natural energies of the sun, moon, earth, stars, and other environmental forces.

The Universal Healing Tao practices are derived from ancient techniques rooted in the processes of nature. They have been gathered and integrated into a coherent, accessible system for well-being that works directly with the life force, or chi, that flows through the meridian system of the body.

Master Chia has spent years developing and perfecting techniques for teaching these traditional practices to students around the world through ongoing classes, workshops, private instruction, and healing sessions, as well as through books and videos and audio products. Further information can be obtained at universal-tao.com.

THE UNIVERSAL HEALING TAO TRAINING CENTER

The Tao Garden Resort and Training Center in northern Thailand is the home of Master Chia and serves as the worldwide headquarters for Universal Healing Tao activities. This integrated wellness, holistic health, and training center is situated on eighty acres surrounded by the beautiful Himalayan foothills, near the historic walled city of Chiang Mai. The serene setting includes flower and herb gardens ideal for meditation, open-air pavilions for practicing Chi Kung, and a health and fitness spa.

The center offers classes year-round, as well as summer and winter retreats. It can accommodate two hundred students, and group leasing can be arranged. For information on courses, books, products, and other resources, see below.

Universal Healing Tao Center
274 Moo 7, Luang Nua, Doi Saket, Chiang Mai, 50220 Thailand
Tel: (66)(53) 921-200
E-mail: universaltao@universal-tao.com
Website: universal-tao.com
For information on retreats and the health spa, contact:
Tao Garden Health Spa & Resort
Website: mantakchia.com/tao-garden

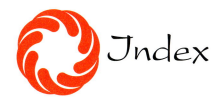

Index

Abdominal Breathing, 8–12, *9*
Activating the Three Fires, 13–16, *13–15*
adrenal gland center, 45
adrenaline, 5
after-birth care, 122–25
aging, 38–43
Agni Yoga, 155
Alchemy of Love, 31–34
amrita, 63
anus, 78, 82–83
anxiety, 92
arousal, 3, 42, 78–79
asexuality, 69
Astral Vertical Flight Training, 148–49
autism, 113

bamboo hitters, 22–25, *24*
Bartholin's glands, 77–78, 79
big toe point, 46
birth, 27, 109
    after-birth care, 122–25
    birthing position and environment, 111–12
    cord-cutting and, 117–22
    importance of the placenta, 112–14
    timing, 110–11
birth trauma, 95–96
black holes, 43
Black Tortoise, 92
bladder, 36
blood circulation, 40
Blue Deer, 92
bonding, 43
bone marrow, 23
bones, 22–25, *24*
breast-feeding, 92–94, 139–45
breast massage, 22
breath and breathing, 3–4, 107, 111
Bubbling Spring point, 46
buffalo yoni, 61
bulban, 66
bulbous glands, 79

Carroll, Lee, 156, 158–59
Castaneda, Carlos, 63
center opposite the heart, 45
cervix, 79
chakras, 40
Charaka Samhita, 64
chi, 4–5, 40

175

176 Index

Chi Kung, 128
Chi Kung Melting Embrace, 153–55
childbirth, 57
Chi Nei Tsang, 55
Chinese medicine, 5
Church, 68–69
clitoris, 63, 77–79, 83
colostrum, 22, 104, 123, 140
communication, 136–39
compassion, 3, 31–32
conception, 3, 21, 27, *58*
  alchemy of, 53–56, 63–65
  water elements and, 65–67
Conception Channel, 43
cord-cutting, 117–22
cosmetic surgery, 67
creativity, 33, 82, 139
crown point, 45
Crystal Palace, 45
C-sections, 95
cyclic breathing, 107

Dadasheva-Drown, Marina
  field notes of, 74, 99–101, 110–11,
    116–17, 118–21, 129–32,
    137–39, 140–41, 144–45, 161
  illustrations of, *26, 52, 84, 108,
    126, 150*
desire, 57
digestion, 4–5
dioxins, 67
DNA, renewal of through sex, 3
dolphins, 66–67, 160–62
Don Juan, 63, 98
Door of Life, 45
Dragon Tears, 34–35
Drown, Colin Campbell, 125–36

earth element, 35, *96*
eggs, 2–3, *58*
Einstein, Albert, 8
ejaculation, 75
elements, balancing, 34–38
elimination, 5
Elixir of Immortality, 38, 61
embryo, 43
emotions, organs and, 35–36
enteric nervous system, 8
epithelium, 22
erection, 75
erogenous zones, 69–70
erotic dance, 54
erotic massage, 74, 82

family care, 127–28
  breast-feeding, 139–45
  communication with your child,
    136–39
  fathers, 134–36
  mothers, 128–32
  potty training, 146–47
  value of play, 148–49
fasciae, 60
fathers, 134–36
feet, 32
female ejaculation, 80–83
feminine exercises
  Ovarian Breathing, 12–13
  Smiling Jade Egg exercise, 17–19
  Warming the Breasts, 10–12, *11*
  Yoni Egg practice, 19–22
fetal development, stages of, 101–7, *102*
fire element, 35, *96*
five elements, 8, 96–97, *97*
Flower of Life, *29*

Index 177

food, artificial, 67
freebirth, 66–67, 80
friction, 75
frigidity, 73–74
Functional Channel. *See* Conception
   Channel

gallbladder, 6, 36
Gate of Life and Death, 44
gazelle yoni, 61
Genaro, 63–64
genetic modifications, 68
Governor Channel, 43
Grof, Stanislav, 95, 97–98, 105–6
G-spot, *62*, 63, 73, 78, 80–83
guilt, 73, 94

happiness, 57
Healing Love, 1–2, 27, 42
health, creating, 1–2
heart, 6, 32, 35, 90
HeartMath Institute, 56, 163–64
Heavenly Pool, 46
hippocampus, 20
homebirth, 104
hormones, 104
Hui Yin, 22, 51, 55–56, 82–83
hypersexuality, 82
hypothalamus, 81–82

Immortal Fetus, 43
immortality, 29, 38–43
Indigo Children, 151–53
   heralding the arrival of, 155–58
   mission of, 158–60
Inner Smile, 35–38, *37*, 86–87, 105
intention, 39

jade egg, 17–19, 54
Jade Pillow, 45
Jade Wand, 54, 75–76

Kama Sutra, 54
Karsai Nei Tsang, 55
Kegel exercises, 81
kidney center, 45
kidneys, 5, 6, 32, 36, 89
kneecap point, 46
knees, 46
Krishna, 64
Kuan Yin, *19*, 35

large intestines, 6, 35
Leonard, Jim, 105–6
Lermontov, Vladimir, 67
letting go, 73
liberation, 101
libido, 40, 73, 101
liver, 6, 33, 36, 89–90
Lotus Birth, 116, 118
Lotus Meditation, 32–34, *33*
love, 162–64
love and trust, instilling, 94–101
lovemaking
   Alchemy of Love, 31–34
   creativity in, 59–65, *60*, *61*, *62*
lower tan tien, 14, 44, 133–34
lower vault, 82–83
lungs, 6, 35, 88–89

mantras, 70–71
Marquez, Gabriel Garcia, 105
marriage rituals, 31
martial arts, 54
Marx, Karl, 152

178 Index

masculine exercises
  Million Dollar Point for Men,
    16–17
  Sending Fire to the Genitals, 10
  Testicle Breathing, 12–13
masturbation, 80
matchmaking, 54
materialism, 31
meditation, 101
Melchizedek, Drunvalo, 56, 155–56
melting embrace, 153–55
men, 75–80, 145–46
Meneghetti, Antonio, 96–97
metal element, 35, 96
Microcosmic Orbit, 22, 31, 43–49,
  48, 50
Microcosmic Orbit for Partners,
  49–51, 50
middle tan tien, 14
middle warmer, 91
mid-eyebrow point, 45–46
Million Dollar Point for Men, 16–17,
  55
miscarriage, 33
Moisture of Joy, 34–35
moksha, 101
mother matrix, 128–32
muscle rings, 78
music
  love ceremonies and, 55
  spiritual, 33

narcissism, 31
nature, 111
navel center, 44
Nei Kung, 23
nervous system, 4–5

nipple massage, 93
nymphomaniac women, 66

Odent, Michel, 65–66, 132, 139
Opening the Lotus, 72
organs, 5–7, 6
  balancing, 34–38
  elements and, 35–36
  emotions and, 6–7
orgasms, 3, 31, 42, 69, 73, 75–80, 75,
  77
Orr, Leonard, 105–6
Osho, 134
Ovarian Breathing, 12–13
Ovary Palace, 44
overpopulation, 64
ovulation, 22
oxytocin, 57, 112

pakua, 134–35, 135
Panchamakara, 55
pancreas, 6, 35
Pandey, Rajbali, 64
PC muscle, 77
Pearce, Joseph Pearce, 42, 94, 99, 129,
  152, 158, 163
pelvic floor, 44
penis, 75–76, 75
perimenopause, 68
perinatal period, 114–17
perineum, 44, 60–61, 78, 82–83
placenta, 112–14, 114
plateau phase, 75–76, 79
play, value of, 148–49
pleasure, 73–74
point opposite the throat, 45
poisons, 67

Index 179

positions, sexual, 60–61
potty training, 146–47
precum. *See* Tears of the Dragon
pregnancy, 85–86
  Inner Smile, 86–87
  instilling love and trust, 94–101
  preparing for breast-feeding, 92–94
  Six Healing Sounds, 86–91
  stages of fetal development, 101–7, *102*
premature ejaculation, 63
prenatal energy, 45
procreation, 57
prostate gland, 76
pubic bone, 15
purity, 65

reincarnation, 38–39
rejuvenating exercises, 7–8
  Abdominal Breathing, 8–12, *9*
  Activating the Three Fires, 13–16, *13–15*
  Million Dollar Point for Men, 16–17
  Ovarian Breathing, 12–13
  Sending Fire to the Genitals, 10
  Testicle Breathing, 12–13
  Warming the Breasts, 10–12, *11*
rituals, Tantric, 69–72
Roerich, Helena, 155–56
Roerich, Nicholas, 155–56

sacred marriage rituals, 31
sacrum, 15, 44–45
Schore, Allan, 99
second brain, 8
Sending Fire to the Genitals, 10

sex and sexuality
  creativity in, 59–65, *60, 61, 62*
  end of, 67–69
  energy of the heart, 56–59
  physiology of, 73–74
sexual center, 44
sexual energy, 5–7, 29–31, *33*
sexual revolution, 67
Shakti, 55
shame, 73, 94
Shiva, 55, 64
Six Healing Sounds, 31, 33, 86–91, 105
Skene's glands, 77, 79, 80
small brain point, 45
small intestines, 6, 35
Smiling Deer, 39–42, *41*
Smiling Jade Egg exercise, 17–19
sodium sulfates, 67–68
solar plexus center, 46
sperm, 2–3, 28, 34–35, *58*
Sperm Palace, 44
spleen, 6, 33, 35, 90–91
squirting, 73, 77, 80–83
sterility, 68
stomach, 35
Svetlana (client), 99–101

Tantra, 54, 69–72
Tao, 5, 57
Tapping for Bone Health, 23–25, *24*
Tears of the Dragon, 55, 63
Testicle Breathing, 12–13
third eye, 45–46
throat point, 46
thumb-sucking, 115
tigress yoni, 61

180 Index

transformative processes, *28*, 29–31

Triple Warmer, 6, 91

ultrasounds, 86, 100

umbilical cord, 115–16, 117–22

unborn children, 85–86

unconditional love, 36–37

upper tan tien, 14

urethral sponge, 78, 79, 80

urinary bladder, 6

urogenital diaphragm, 63

uterus, 11

vagina, 60–63, *62*, 76–78, *77*

Verny, Thomas, 85–86

Vishnu, 64

Warming the Breasts, 10–12, *11*, 92

water, 105, 122–23

water birth, 80

water element, 35, 36, 65–67, 96

weaning, 144–45

whales, 66

White Tantra, 55

women

  exercises, 10–12, 12–13, 17–19, 19–22

  orgasm and, 75–80

  physiology of sex and, 73–74

  restrictions on, 69

wood element, 36, 96

Wu Chi, *30*

yang, 6, 43, 65, 96

Yang Channel, 43

Yellow Emperor, 40, 54, 158

Yellow Phoenix, 92–93, *93*

yin, 6, 43, 65, 96

yoni, 60–63, *62*

Yoni Egg practice, 19–22, 81

zygote, 98